ARCHERY ANATOMY

ARCHERY ANATOMY

An Introduction to Techniques for Improved Performance

Ray Axford

SOUVENIR PRESS

First published 1995 by Souvenir Press Limited,
43 Great Russell Street, London WC1B 3PA
and simultaneously in Canada.

ISBN 0 285 63265 6

Typeset by Rowland Phototypesetting Limited,
Bury St Edmunds, Suffolk.
Printed in Great Britain by
St Edmundsbury Press Limited,
Bury St Edmunds, Suffolk.

Author's Note

Although *Archery Anatomy* is intended as a primer of anatomical biomechanics and elementary physical mechanics as they relate to archery, it assumes that the reader will be familiar with the practice and/or instruction of a basic archery shooting technique as covered by the majority of national coaching manuals.

The anatomical names of muscles and bones used throughout the book are mainly those of the Basel Terminology, as revised and corrected by the 5th and 6th International Congress of Anatomists.

Contents

Sighters

Seeing the objective

The ideal archer should have a complete shooting technique that is simple and uncomplicated; all movements and action should be performed smoothly and naturally, the body and bow moving and working together as one familiar unit. The whole archer, from head to feet, will be composed and balanced with no unnecessary tension in any area; mentally and physically relaxed, but alert.

In coming to full draw, the whole body should aim naturally in the direction of the target, in such a way that if the draw were executed and completed with the eyes closed, upon opening the eyes to confirm the aim, it would only be necessary to adjust the angle of trajectory vertically, with little or no adjustment of direction laterally.

The head should neither hinder nor compromise the development of an anatomically efficient draw. The structure of the face and the lower jaw should be used only to position the controlling aiming eye consistently behind the bow string at a fixed height and attitude above the arrow nock, to confirm that the aim of body and bow is correct; the brain within will meanwhile monitor and confirm, by the feel of the body actions and loads, that the sequence has been and will be efficiently completed. All body actions, movements and positions will, where possible, take advantage of any unavoidable loads imposed by the natural laws of physics to minimise the expenditure of energy; there should be no conflict between the efficient use of mind and body and the demands required to exploit the efficiency of the equipment.

Archery, along with other closed or open motor skill sports, relies very much on mental concentration, determination, motivation and visualisation, and considerable emphasis has quite rightly been placed upon the mental approach to sports training and performance.

However, no sport can rely upon mental powers alone. The efficient physical application of the bones, joints, tendons and muscles of the body must also be examined, understood and applied to obtain the best performance from each individual. The mental requirements are then supported and given greater meaning, while self-confidence, enjoyment, competitiveness and mental relaxation are also improved and developed.

The archer opposite may be assumed to display many of the physical ideals and to possess all the mental requirements. In the following pages, certain areas of the archer and equipment will be examined in some detail and the loaded actions of body and bow will be analysed to determine whether the existing or intended technique could be performed more efficiently.

NOTE: Sighters are six arrows shot at the start of a round, to check that the body and equipment are correctly prepared and fit for the work to come.

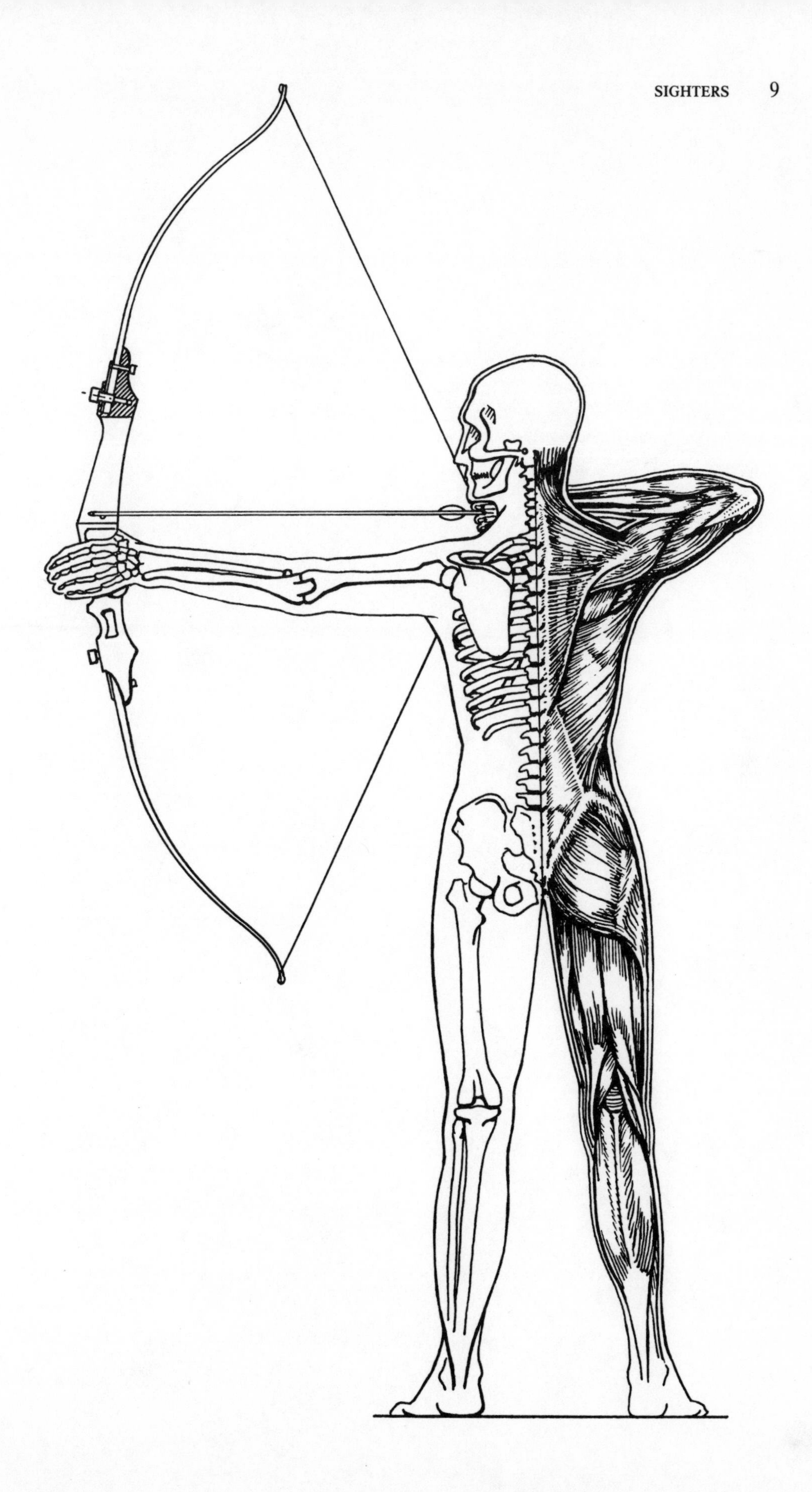

PART ONE

BODY AND BOW ANATOMY

1 Human Body Anatomy

GENERAL DESCRIPTION

Knowledge of the anatomical structure of the human body is essential if the efficient application of its use is to be fully appreciated.

The skeleton, with an average dry weight of 8½ lbs (3.86 kilos) is the firm, bony framework of the human body. It constitutes partly a support of compressive loads and partly a protective cover of the inner organs.

The individual bones are linked together in different ways, and these joints may be movable or immovable. The joints we are concerned with are mainly movable.

The majority of the 233 bones of the skeleton are symmetrical handed pairs, while the single bones, such as the vertebrae and pelvis, are composed of two similar subdivisions.

In movable joints the contacting surfaces of the bones are covered with cartilage and their strongest connecting elements are the capsular ligaments that hold the joint together. The forms of the articulating surfaces of the joints determine the function and may be flat, spherical, cylindrical, screwlike or saddle-shaped.

When moved, the bones generally act as levers rotating around an imaginary axis; they are moved by muscles connected at one end to the bone to be moved via a tendon, and at the other via a tendon to the supporting structure.

When a given joint is in a position where the muscles controlling it are relaxed or in a state of equal minimum contraction, the joint is said to be in a state of rest. This is the starting point of every analysis of joint movement.

NOTE: It is more important to know where the muscles are which perform the actions of bones and joints, and their location in relation to the bones and joints, so that they can be identified by feel and observation, than to know every bone, muscle and joint by name. However, to be able to name them in correspondence and telephone conversations is an asset to both sides.

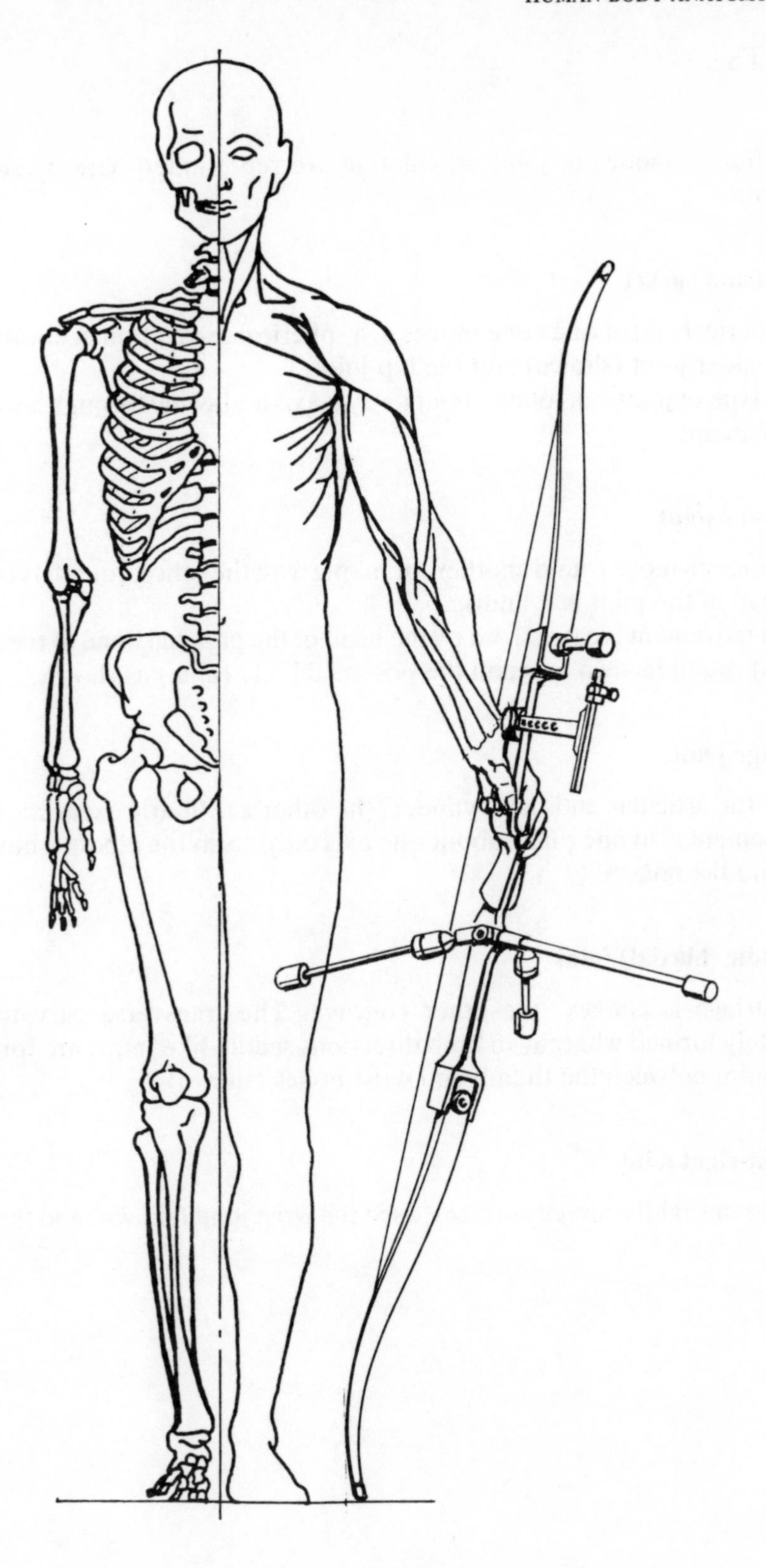

JOINTS

The different modes of joint articulation are represented here by schematic diagrams.

1 Ball and socket

The spherical end of one bone moves in a spherical excavation in another, as in the shoulder joint (shown) and the hip joint.

This type of joint can rotate about its own axis and swing through a wide cone of movement.

2 Rotary joint

One bone can move round another, or, along with the other, round its own axis. The head of the joint is cylindric.

Such movement is carried out by the head of the preaxial bone of the forearm (radius) round its own axis and the postaxial bone (ulna) as shown.

3 Hinge joint

One of the articular ends is a cylinder, the other a cylindric excavation.

Movement is in one plane about one axis only, as in the elbow (shown), the knee and the fingers.

4 Saddle (biaxial) joint

One surface is convex, the other concave. The transverse curvatures are oppositely formed whereby in both directions saddle-like joints are formed, as in the joint between the thumb and wrist bones (shown).

5 Semi-rigid joint

With flat or slightly curved surfaces, as in the wrist joint (shown) and the instep.

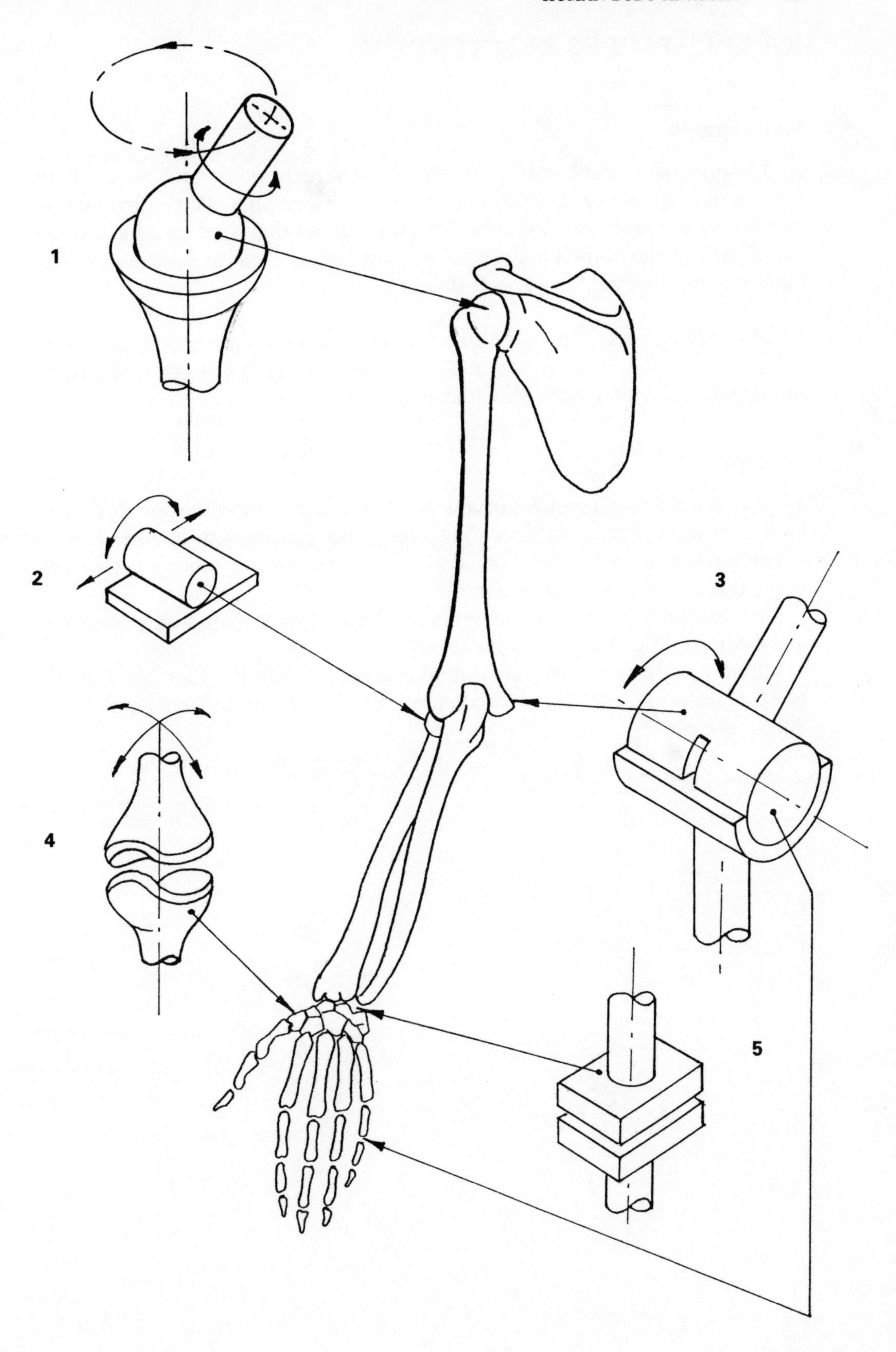
1
2
3
4
5

JOINT CAPSULES AND TENDONS

Joint capsules

1 The majority of limb joints are synovial—where the ends of the bones are in contact they are covered with a special articular cartilage. The entire joint is covered by a capsule lined with synovial membrane that secretes a lubricating fluid. The capsule of the joint is reinforced in certain areas by ligaments which hold the joint together and give it stability.

2 The encapsulated joint may also contain ligaments within it, as in the case of the knee, or other structures such as the long head of the biceps tendon and supraspinatus tendon in the shoulder joint (shown).

Tendons

3 Tendons are tough bundles of collagen fibres that connect the muscles to the bones, so that muscle contraction pulls the bone, causing movement.

The tendons are attached at one end by the musculo-tendinous junction and at the other by the bony insertion.

Each tendon is covered by a membrane called the paratenon which nourishes and lubricates the tendon to some extent.

Where tendons pass over or around a bone, as with the long head of the biceps tendon in the shoulder, the tendon is further protected and guided by a fibrous sheath.

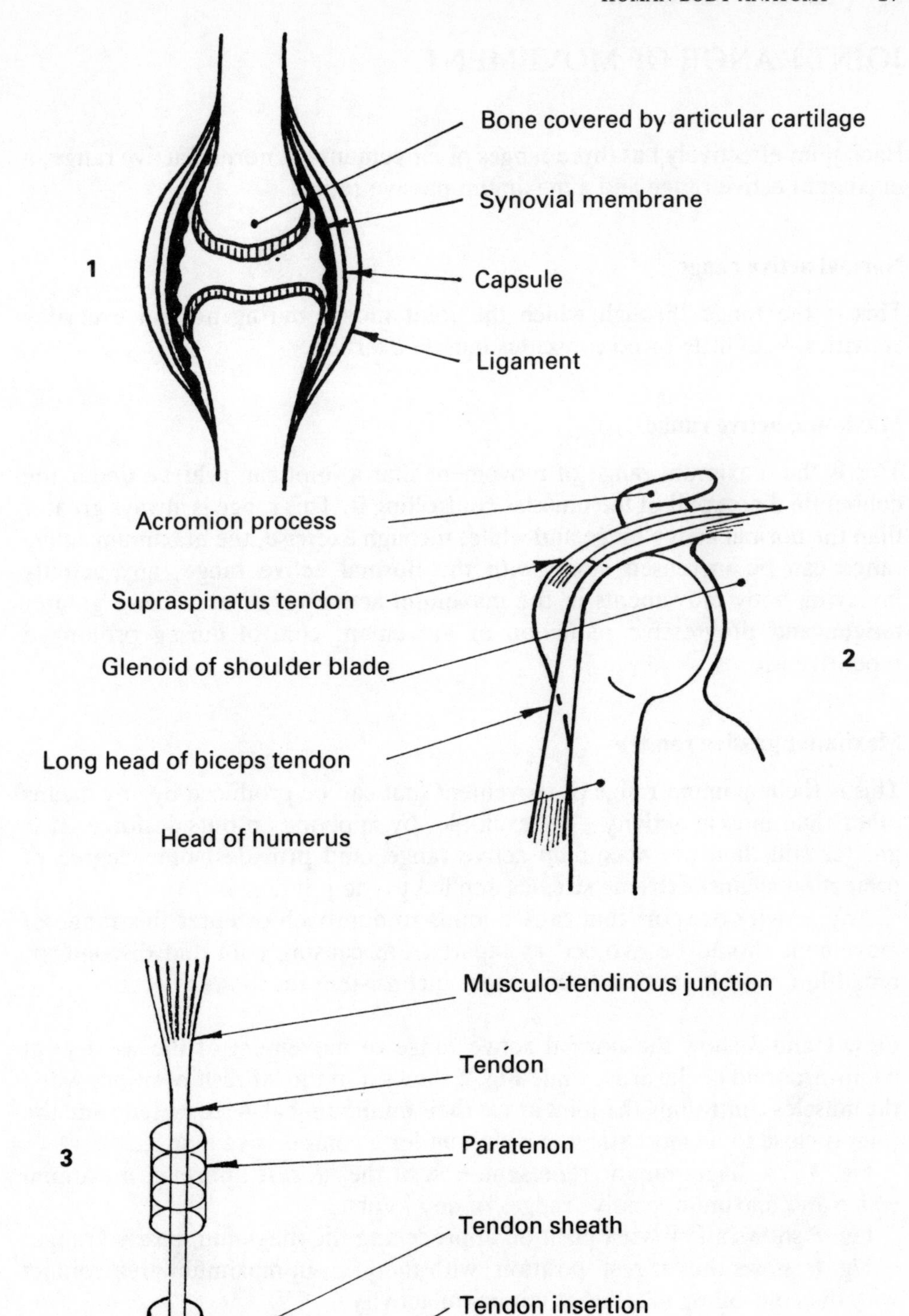
1
Bone covered by articular cartilage
Synovial membrane
Capsule
Ligament
2
Acromion process
Supraspinatus tendon
Glenoid of shoulder blade
Long head of biceps tendon
Head of humerus
3
Musculo-tendinous junction
Tendon
Paratenon
Tendon sheath
Tendon insertion

JOINT RANGE OF MOVEMENT

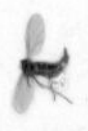

Each joint effectively has three ranges of movement—a normal active range, a maximum active range and a maximum passive range.

Normal active range

This is the range through which the joint moves during normal everyday activities, with little or no conscious muscle exertion.

Maximum active range

This is the maximum range of movement that a joint can achieve under the deliberate direct pull of the muscles controlling it. This range is always greater than the normal active range and while, through exercise, the maximum active range can be increased along with the normal active range, any activity involving body movements in the maximum active range may cause greater fatigue and progressive reduction of movement control during prolonged repetitive use.

Maximum passive range

This is the maximum range of movement that can be produced by any means other than muscle activity—for example, by applying an outside force. It is greater still than the maximum active range, and provides some degree of protection against extreme stresses applied to the joint.

Any activity or sport that causes joints to approach or enter this range of movement should be avoided as, apart from causing pain and discomfort, repetition of such physical stress causes inconsistent reactions to occur.

Figs. 1 and **3** show the normal active range of movement of the wrist joint palmwards and backwards, while **Fig. 2** shows it in the 'at rest' position, when the muscles controlling the joint are at their minimum balanced activity and the joint is close to its most stable position under a compressive load.

Fig. 4 is a diagrammatic representation of the 'at rest', normal, maximum active and maximum passive ranges of any joint.

Fig. 5 shows a low wrist position approaching the maximum passive range.

Fig. 6 shows the 'at rest' position, with the joint in maximum area contact with the controlling muscles at minimum activity.

Fig. 7 illustrates the high wrist position, approaching the maximum passive range.

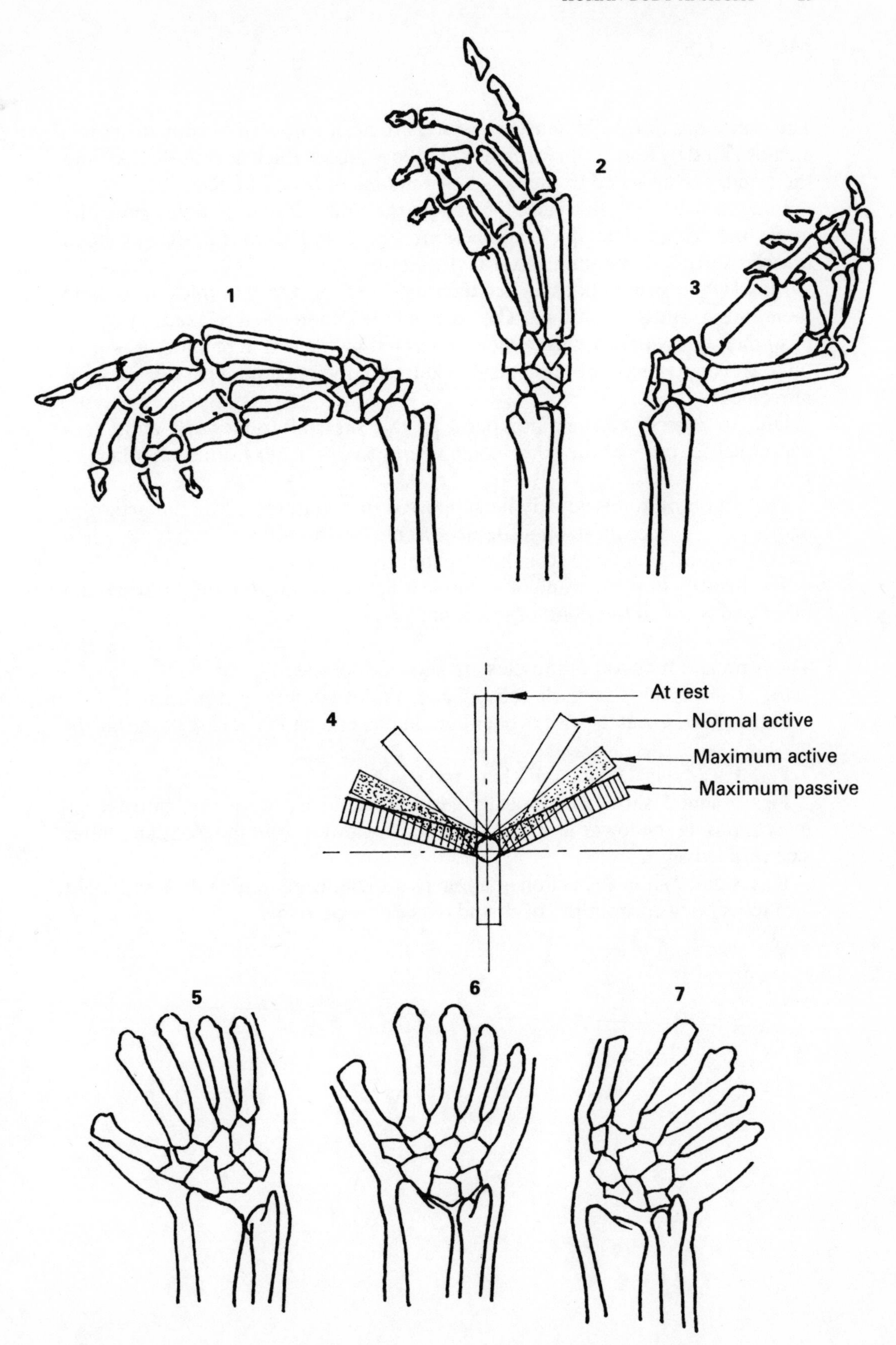
1
2
3
4
At rest
Normal active
Maximum active
Maximum passive
5
6
7

MUSCLES

The bones are moved by muscles, which are flesh-coloured fibrous structures encapsulated by fasciae. In form they are long, broad, thick or ring-shaped, and their ends are attached to the bones by tendons or broad fasciae.

Long muscles are, as a rule, located on the limbs. Broad muscles generally move the trunk. The thick muscles are short and powerful. Ring-shaped muscles surround openings, such as the mouth.

Muscles perform actions by contracting: they shorten and thicken, pulling their ends towards each other. They can only lengthen when relaxed, so do not push their ends apart but have them separated by the action of another muscle pulling in opposition or by an outside load, as in the maximum passive range of movement.

Due to muscle contraction, parts of the skeletal framework and, as a consequence, parts of the body, come nearer to or farther from each other, or rotate.

The action of a muscle may be supported or counteracted by the action of another. As a rule, these opposite actions are performed alternately, as when the limbs bend (flex) and straighten (extend).

The fixed or stationary end of a muscle is called the head or origin, while the other end is called the point of insertion.

The form and function of muscles are shown opposite.

Fig. 1 shows a long muscle relaxed and, in dotted outline, contracted.

Fig. 2 shows a muscle with two tendons at one end, as in the case of the biceps muscle.

Fig. 3 is a typical broad muscle of the trunk.

Figs. 4 and **5** show anatomically and schematically the action of a biceps muscle raising the lower arm lever (right arm viewed from the front and inner side respectively).

Figs. 6 and **7** show the action of a triceps muscle straightening the lower right arm lever, viewed from the back and outside respectively.

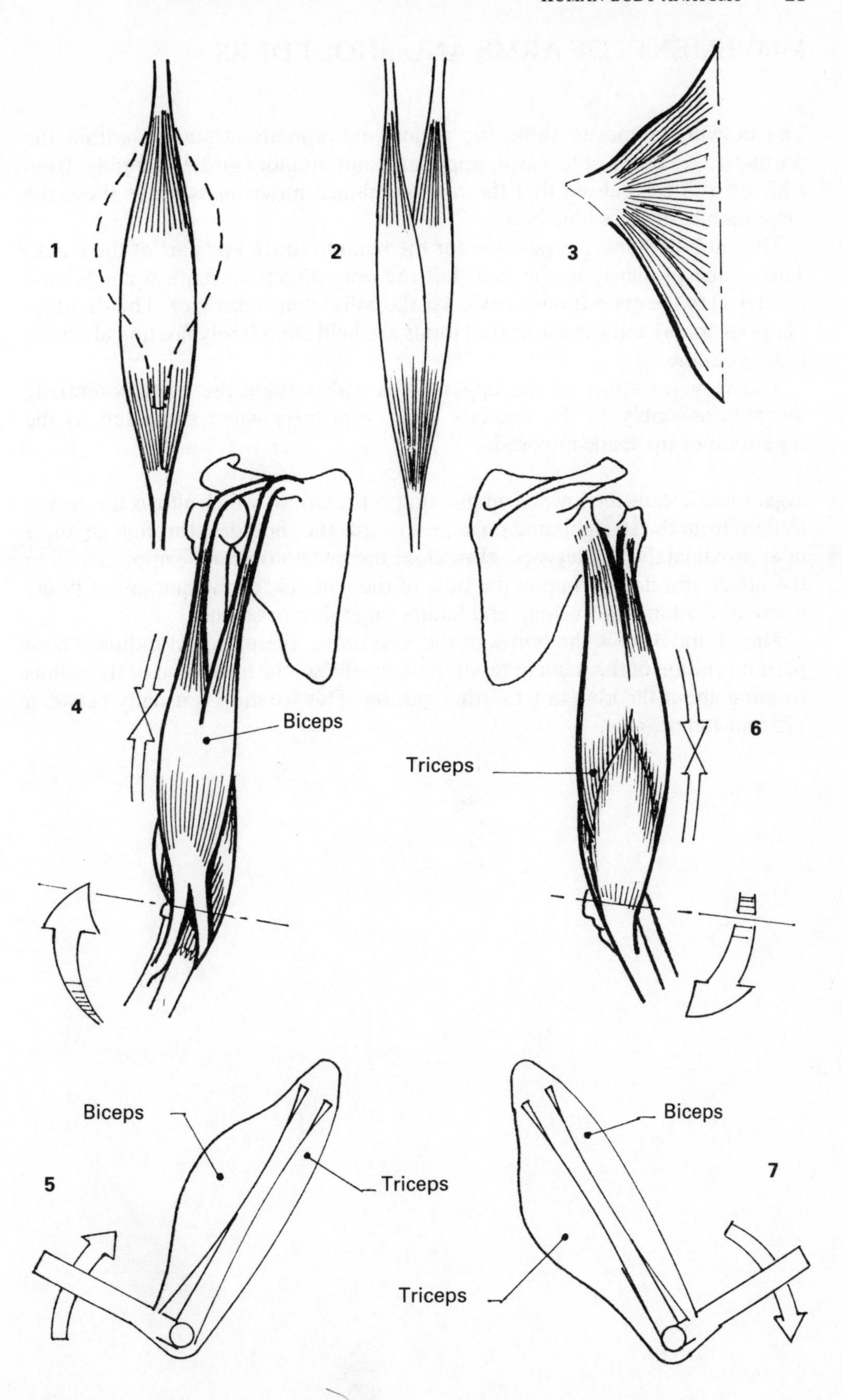
1
2
3
4
Biceps
Triceps
6
Biceps
5
Triceps
Biceps
7
Triceps

MOVEMENTS OF ARMS AND SHOULDERS

The drawings opposite show the various movements attainable within the normal active range of forearm, upper arm and shoulder girdle assembly, from which it will be realised that the total combined movements make these the most mobile of the whole body.

This mobility makes it possible for the hand to touch any part of the trunk. This is due primarily to the fact that the only direct mechanical connection (skeletal) to the main framework is via the collar bone (clavicle). The shoulder blade (scapula) and the associated joints are held from freely floating about by muscles alone.

The very versatility of the upper limbs makes them the most potentially unstable assembly of the archer's body, especially when subjected to the repetition of the loads imposed.

Figs. 1 and **2** show the lower arm pivoting at the elbow, which allows the arm to fold up from the straightened position towards the shoulder, through an angle of approximately 156 degrees. How close the lower arm can be approached to the upper arm depends upon the bulk of the muscles, or the amount of fleshy tissue or clothing intervening and hampering this movement.

Figs. 1 and **3** show the bones of the lower arm, the ulna and radius. These permit rotation of the hand in relation to the elbow, the lower end of the radius rotating about the ulna in a twisting motion. This rotation is usually between 170 and 180 degrees.

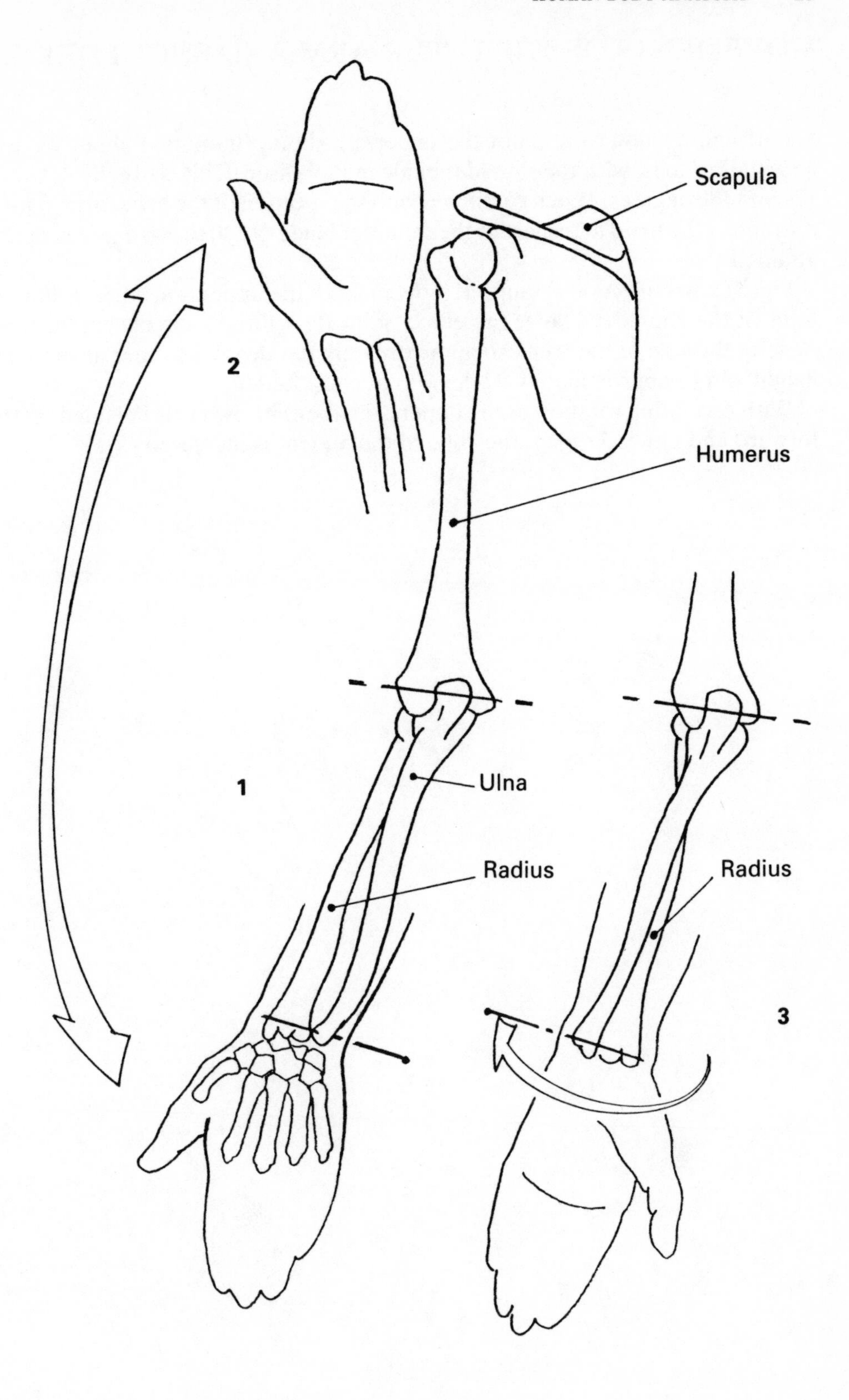
Scapula
2
Humerus
1
Ulna
Radius
Radius
3

MOVEMENTS OF THE UPPER ARM AND SHOULDER

Figs. 1 and **2** show rotation of the upper arm bone (humerus) about its own longitudinal axis, with the shoulder blade immobilised. This is usually between 170 and 180 degrees. When combined with the rotation of the lower arm, a total rotation of the hand in respect to the shoulder blade of 340 to 360 degrees can be attained.

Fig. 3 shows the conical range of movement of the upper arm bone within the joint of the shoulder blade, the elbow joint describing a circular path, from close to the side of the trunk to approximately ten degrees to rear at shoulder height and to approximately 90 degrees at chest height.

With oscillating rotation of the upper arm about its own axis included on the forward and upward swing, the cone of movement is increased.

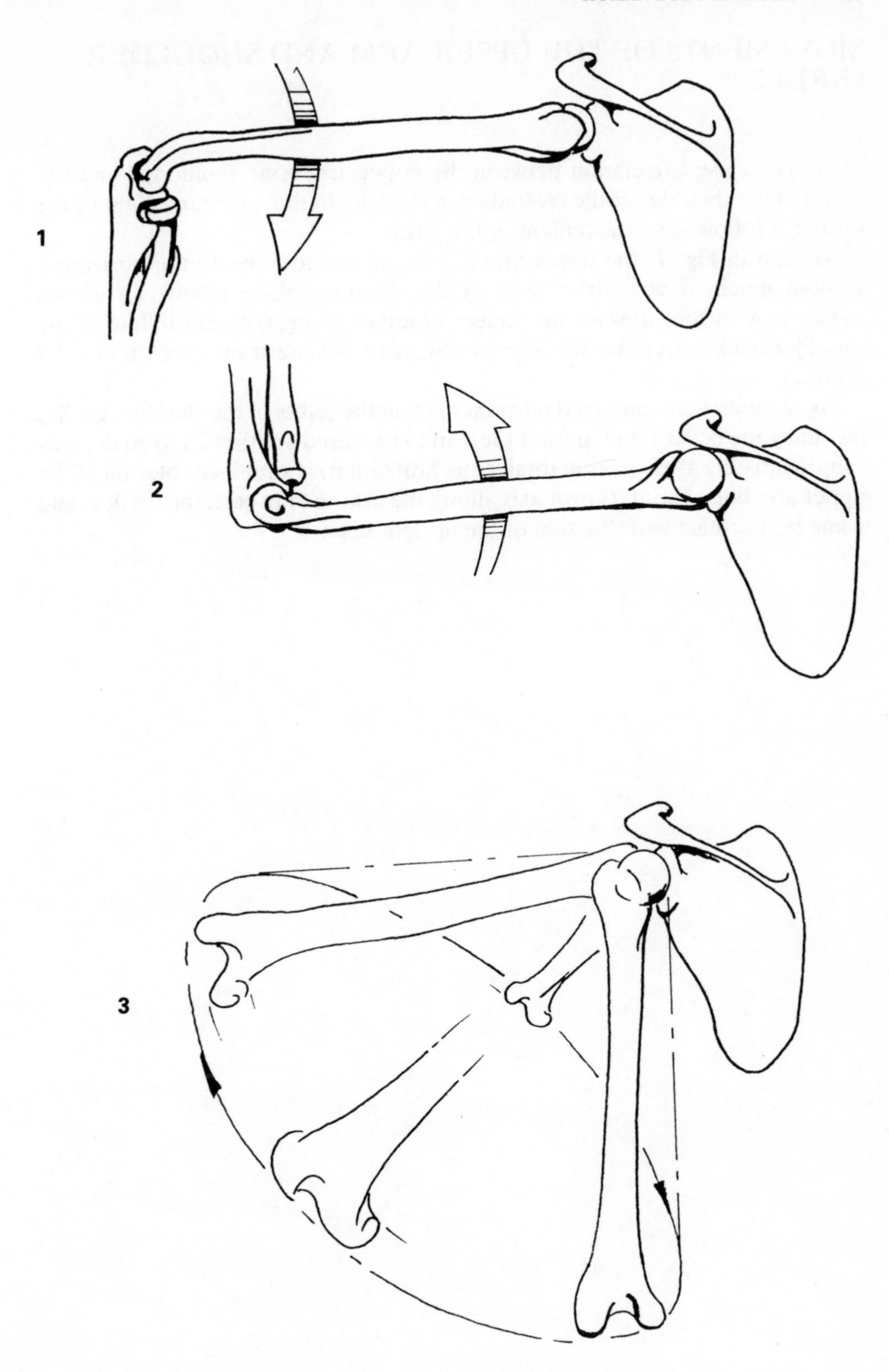
1
2
3

MOVEMENTS OF THE UPPER ARM AND SHOULDER GIRDLE

There is a close correlation between the upper arm bone (humerus) and the bones of the shoulder girdle (scapula and clavicle) in that any movement of the former is followed by movement of the latter.

As seen in **Fig. 1**, the upper arm can be raised sideways to the horizontal without much, if any, movement of the shoulder blade (shown in dotted outline). A further upward movement of about 20 degrees can follow as the shoulder blade moves upwards and outwards from the trunk (shown in solid outline).

Fig. 2 shows that combined movement of all the joints of the shoulder girdle, including the collar bone, permit the arm to be raised another 25 to 30 degrees (approximately 45 degrees in total to the horizontal). Combined rotation of the upper arm bone about its own axis allows the arm to approach the vertical and come into contact with the side of the upright head.

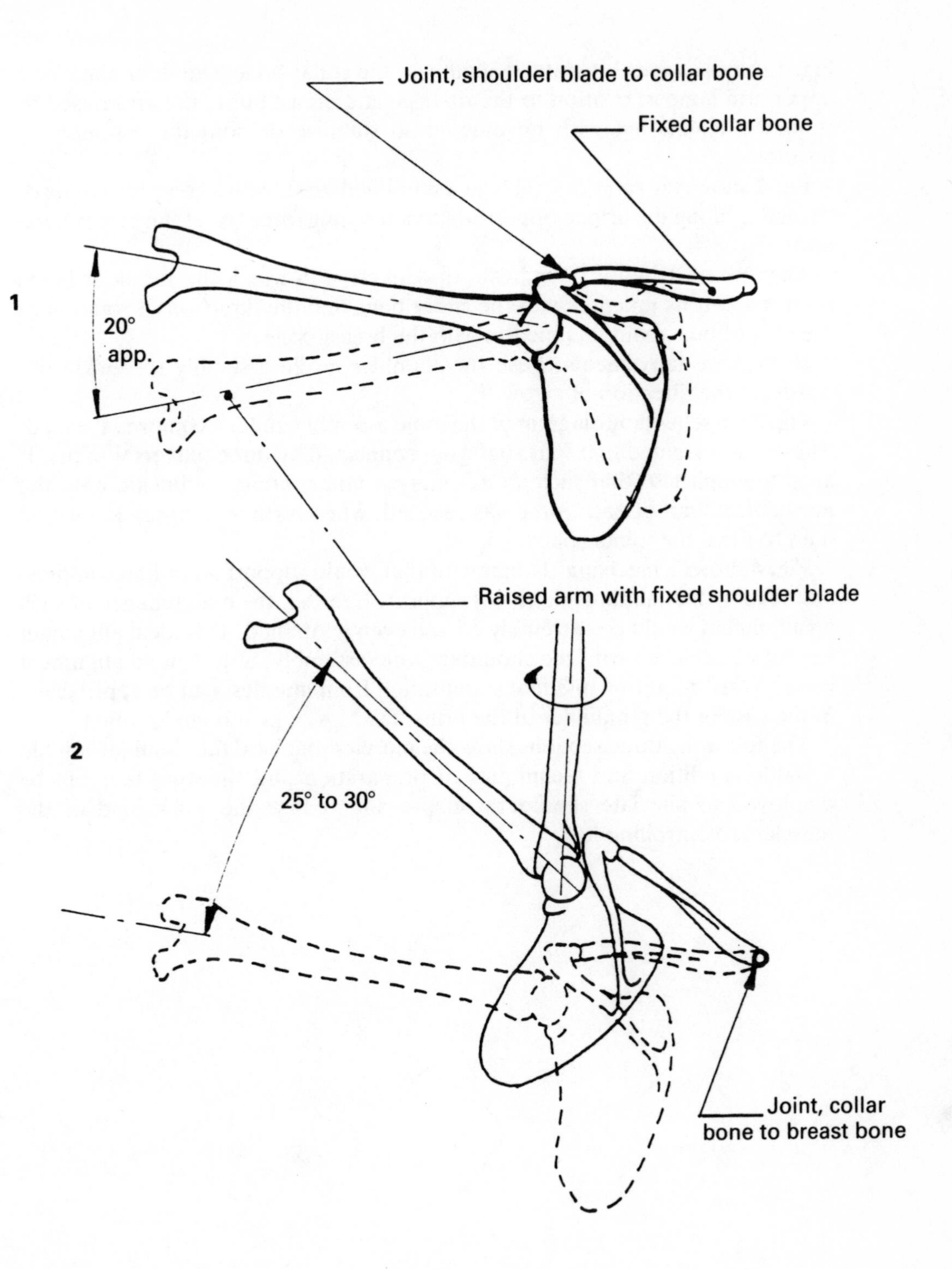
Joint, shoulder blade to collar bone
Fixed collar bone
1
20°
app.
Raised arm with fixed shoulder blade
2
25° to 30°
Joint, collar
bone to breast bone

MECHANICAL ALIGNMENT OF THE UPPER ARM AND SHOULDER GIRDLE

Fig. 1 shows a typical skeletal assembly of the collar bone, shoulder blade and upper arm bone in relation to the rib cage and breast bone, the arm raised to shoulder height, but with no muscles to stabilise or hold the assembly in position.

Fig. 2 shows the same assembly in a simplified form, with a compressive force 'B' acting along the arm in opposition to a resisting force 'A' at the breast bone joint.

The arrows 'C' and 'D' indicate the direction in which the shoulder blade rotates about its junction with the collar bone and the direction of rotation of the collar bone about its junction with the breast bone.

Both these movements cause the shoulder girdle assembly to buckle upwards, in the direction of arrow 'E'.

Fig. 3 is a schematic diagram of the same assembly under a compressive load, where it is imagined that four shafts are connected by three universal joints. It aims to emphasise that such an assembly would continue to buckle until the mechanical limit of each joint was reached, when further compression would tend to force the joints apart.

Fig. 4 shows a mechanical alignment that would support an in-line compressive load with minimum additional support. Even so, the maintenance of such an alignment would be extremely critical even if attained. This ideal alignment cannot be achieved with the shoulder girdle assembly, although an alignment close to this, requiring minimal stabilisation from muscles, can be approached in the case of the remainder of the arms, the hips, legs and ankle joints.

The following three sections show the muscles that hold the shoulder joint in a stable condition and techniques of preparation and shooting that can be employed to alleviate shoulder collapse and reduce the work load of the muscles in controlling it.

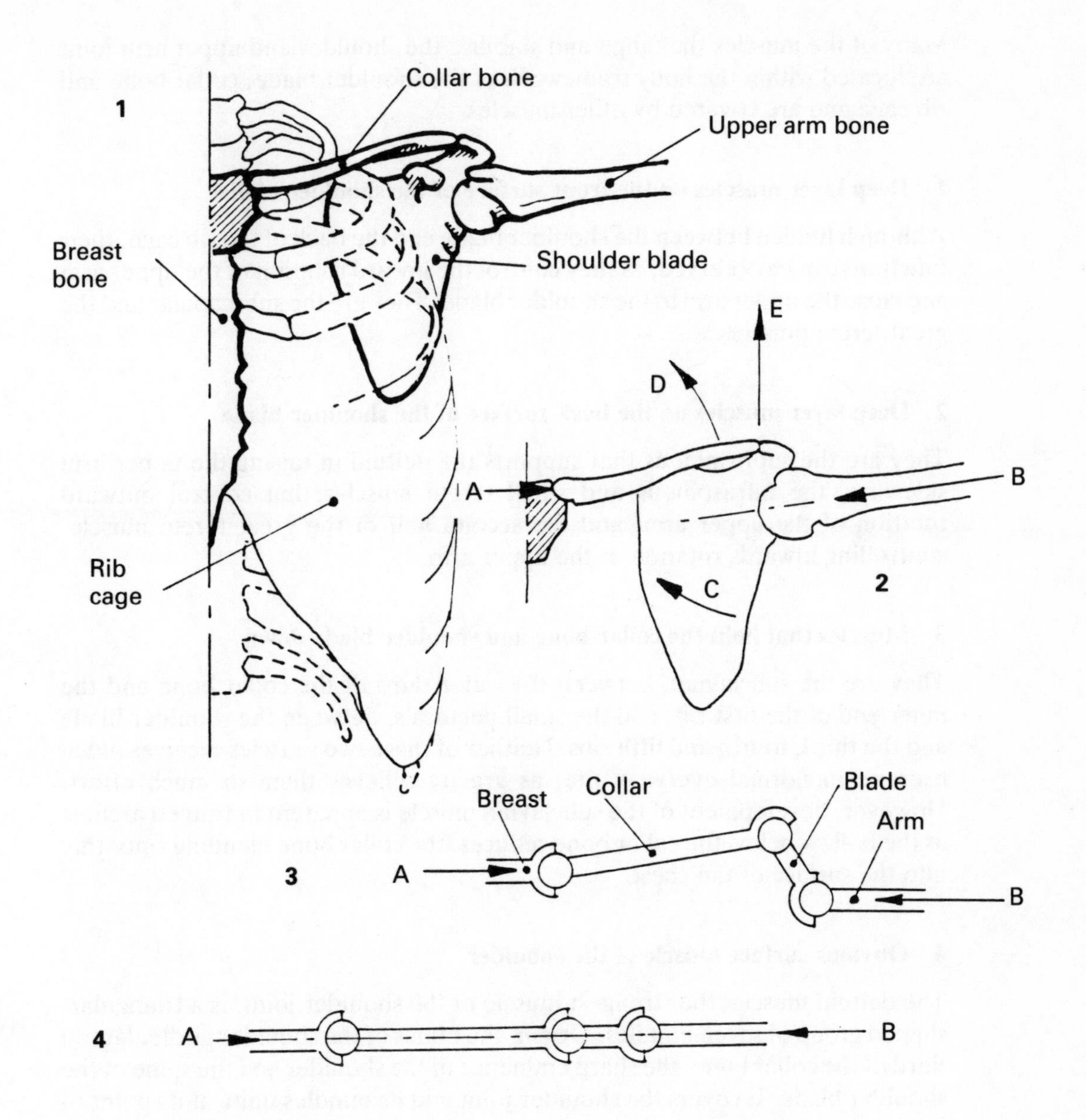
1
Collar bone
Upper arm bone
Breast bone
Shoulder blade
Rib cage
E
D
A
B
C
2
Breast
Collar
Blade
Arm
3
A
B
4
A
B

MUSCLES OF THE SHOULDER

Many of the muscles that align and stabilise the shoulder and upper arm joint are located within the bony framework of the shoulder blade, collar bone and rib cage and are covered by other muscles.

1 Deep layer muscles on the front surface of the shoulder blade

Although hidden between the shoulder blade and the back of the rib cage, their functions can be observed, as they control the inward rotation of the upper arm and close the upper arm to the shoulder blade. They are the subscapular and the great terete muscles.

2 Deep layer muscles on the back surface of the shoulder blade

They are the supraspinous that supports the deltoid in raising the upper arm sideways; the infraspinous and small terete muscles that control outward rotation of the upper arm; and the second half of the great terete muscle, controlling inwards rotation of the upper arm.

3 Muscles that hold the collar bone and shoulder blade down

They are the subclavian, between the outer third of the collar bone and the inner end of the first rib, and the small pectorals, between the shoulder blade and the third, fourth and fifth ribs. Neither of these two muscles receives much exercise in normal everyday life, as gravity relieves them of much effort. However, development of the subclavian muscle is apparent in trained archers as the hollow below the collar bone reduces, the collar bone blending smoothly into the surface of the chest.

4 Obvious surface muscle of the shoulder

The deltoid muscle, the strongest muscle of the shoulder joint, is a triangular-shaped group of seven bundles. Origin, the bones of the shoulder girdle, lateral third of the collar bone, the sharp eminence of the shoulder and the spine of the shoulder blade. It covers the shoulder joint and its bundles unite at its point of insertion to the upper arm bone midway between the shoulder and elbow joints on the outer surface.

Contraction of the whole muscle raises the arm sideways to the horizontal position in respect to the shoulder blade, partial contraction of the back or front part give a backwards or forwards movement of the arm.

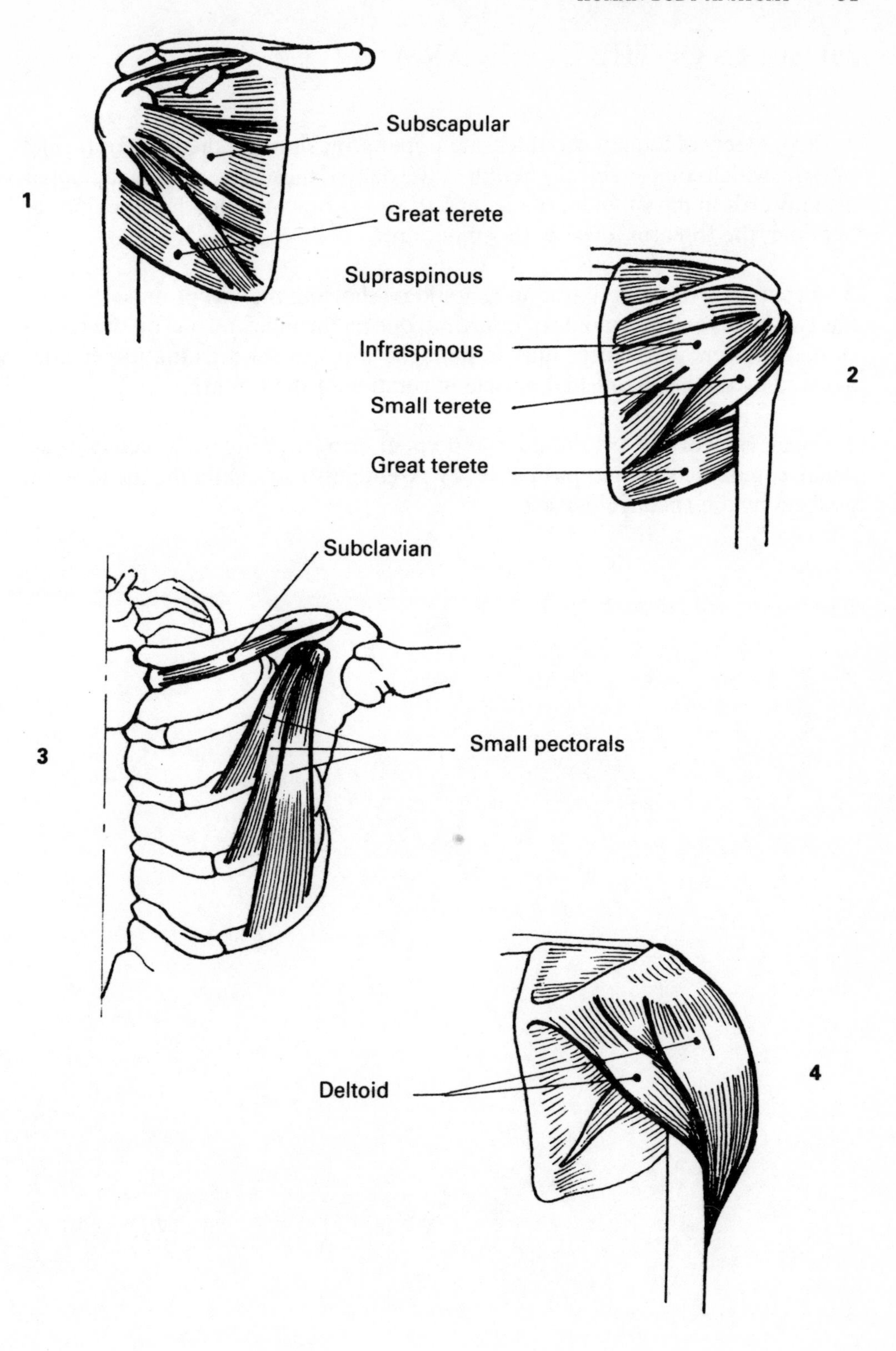
Subscapular
1
Great terete
Supraspinous
Infraspinous
2
Small terete
Great terete
Subclavian
3
Small pectorals
Deltoid
4

MUSCLES OF THE UPPER ARM

1 Front view of the left shoulder and upper arm, showing the coracobrachial muscle, which counteracts the action of the deltoid muscle by pulling the upper arm inwards to the shoulder blade, and the inner brachial muscle in flexion, or bending, the forearm towards the upper arm.

2 Front view of the left arm and shoulder, showing the biceps muscle which has two heads and two points of insertion, one on the ulna and one on the radius of the forearm. The biceps muscle pulls the forearm towards the upper arm, assisted by the inner brachial muscle in rotation of the forearm.

3 Back view of the left shoulder and upper arm, showing the triceps muscle which counteracts the biceps muscle, by extending or straightening the forearm assisted by the anconeal muscle.

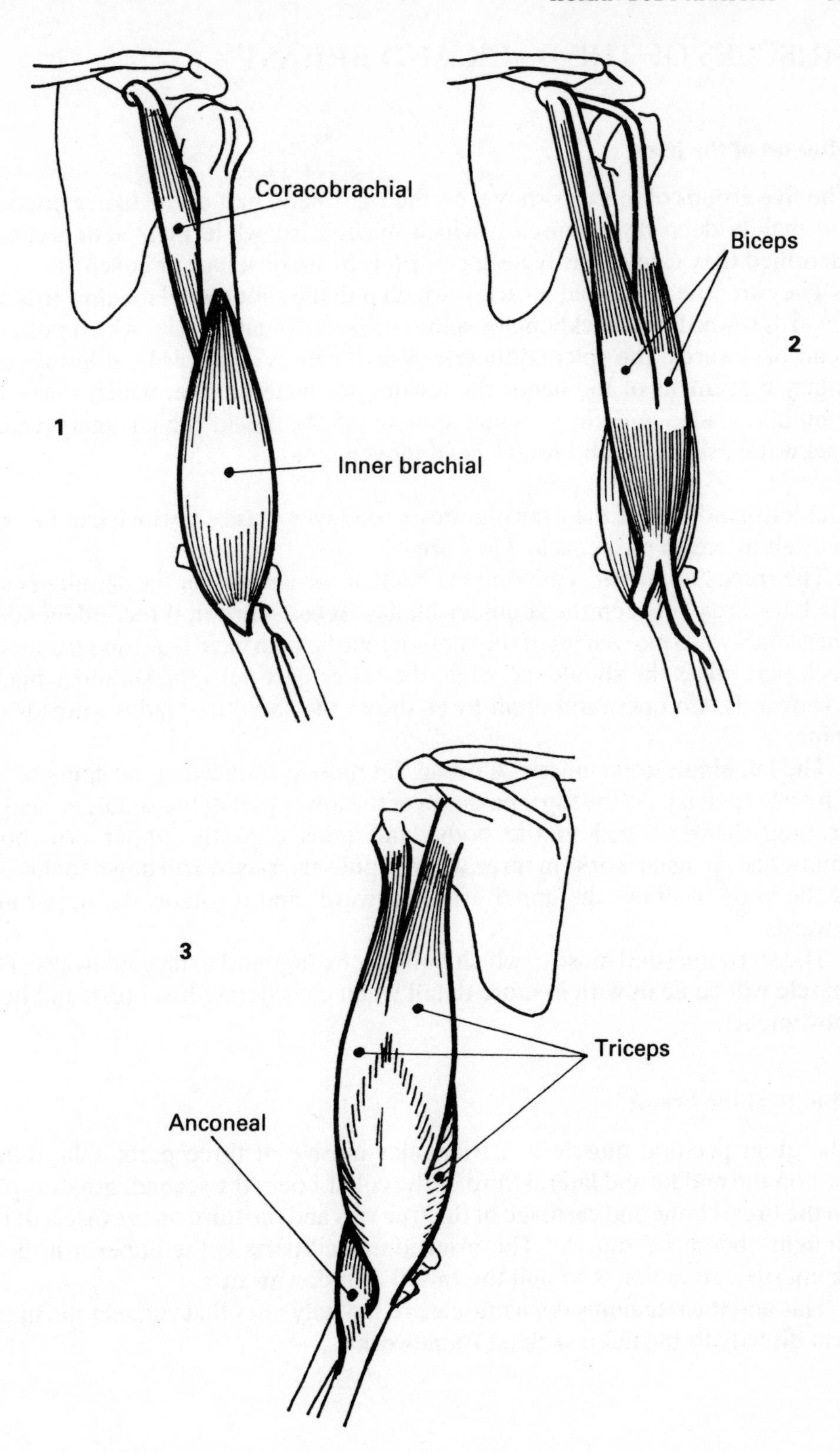
Coracobrachial
1
Inner brachial
Biceps
2
3
Triceps
Anconeal

MUSCLES OF THE BACK AND BREAST

Muscles of the back

The five groups of muscles shown on the right-hand half of the figure opposite are mainly deep layer muscles, which means that while their action can be identified they cannot easily be seen or felt by an observer or coach.

They are: the rhomboid muscles, which pull the shoulder blade upwards and inwards towards the backbone or spine; the semispinal muscle, which pulls the head backwards; the splenial muscle, which causes backwards, sideways and rotary movement of the head; the levator scapulae muscle, which raises the shoulder blade; and the splenial muscle of the neck, which again causes backwards, sideways and rotary head movements.

The left-hand half of the drawing shows top layer muscles, which can be seen and felt in action by a coach. They are:

The trapezius muscle, covering the back of the neck, over the shoulders and the back area between the shoulder blades. It can work in three independent parts: backward movement of the shoulder girdle with fixed head and trunk, the neck part raises the shoulders, while the lower part pulls the shoulder blades downwards. Co-operation of all three draws the shoulder blades towards the spine.

The latissimus dorsi muscle, a broad flat muscle connecting the spine to the hip bone (pelvis). At the top it passes over the lower part of the shoulder blades, keeping them pressed to the body, and joins onto the upper arm bone (humerus). It again works in three ways: it pulls the raised arm down to the side of the body, it draws the upper arm backwards and it rotates the upper arm inwards.

The sternomastoid muscle, which pulls the head round to face sideways. This muscle will be dealt with in more detail when considering head turn and head movements.

Muscle of the breast

The great pectoral muscle is a triangular muscle of three parts—the minor part on the middle and lateral third of the collar bone, the second, greater, part on the breast bone and cartilage of the true ribs and the third on the fascia of the straight abdominal muscle. The insertion of all parts is the upper arm bone (humerus). Its action is to pull the raised arm downwards.

This and the latissimus dorsi muscle are the only ones that connect the upper arm directly to the main skeletal framework.

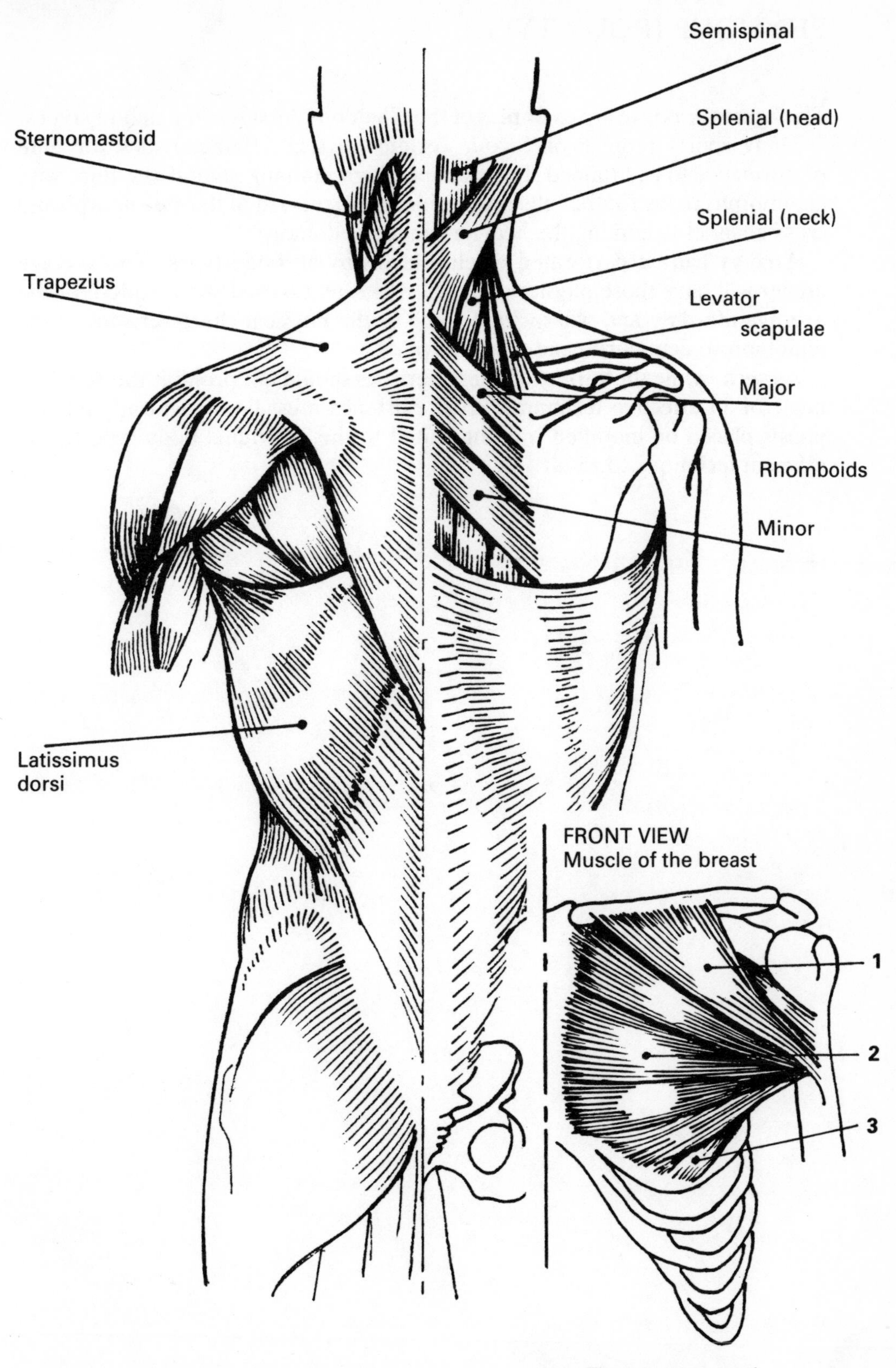

The great pectoral

PHYSIQUE (BODY TYPE)

The figures opposite are examples of the 'Sheldon Classification' of body types.

Many sports require or favour certain physical characteristics for elite performance to be attained. For example, high jumping favours the slim, wiry ectomorph, rugby football the muscle bulk and strength of the mesomorph and cross-channel swimming the heavier-limbed endomorph.

Archery can be performed to elite levels by all body types. The average archer will have those physical characteristics generalised and adapted for the average life-style and will include some of the physical characteristics of the endomorph, ectomorph and mesomorph.

As such, while the variety of characteristics should not prohibit the development of an effective technique, their existence must be recognised and emphasis placed on modified training suited to the individual body type for an efficient technique to result.

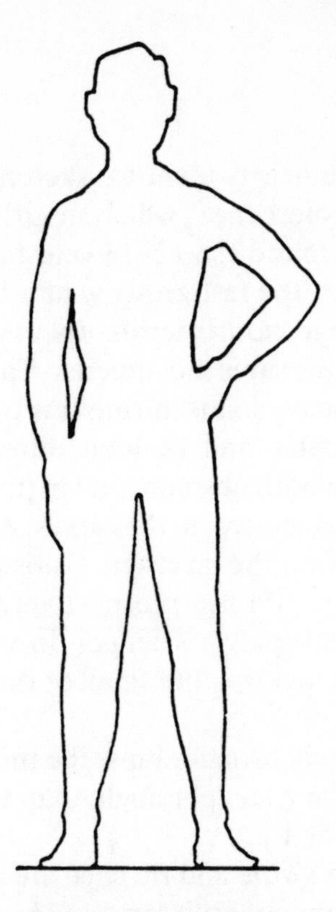

Average physique

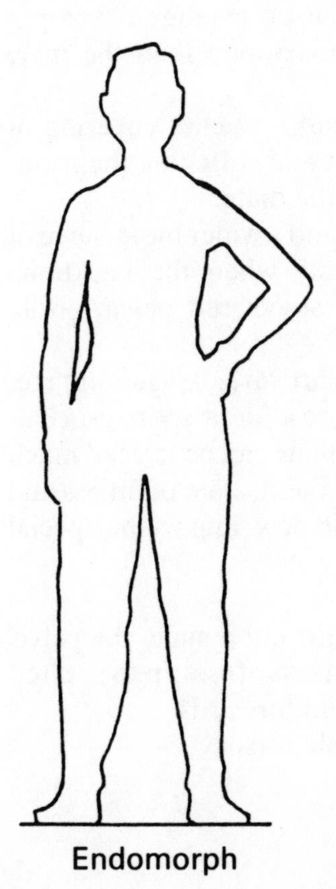

Endomorph

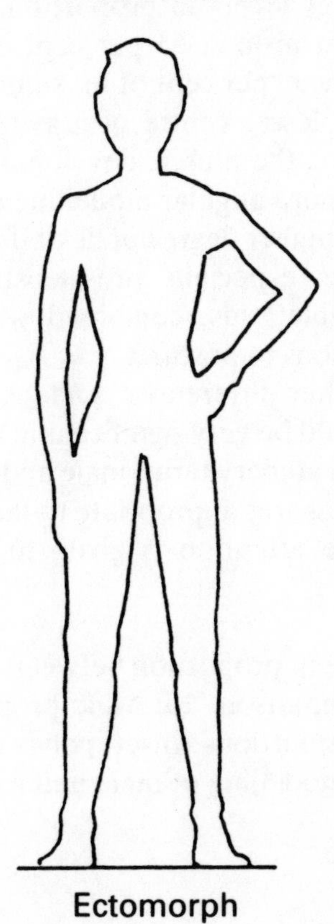

Ectomorph

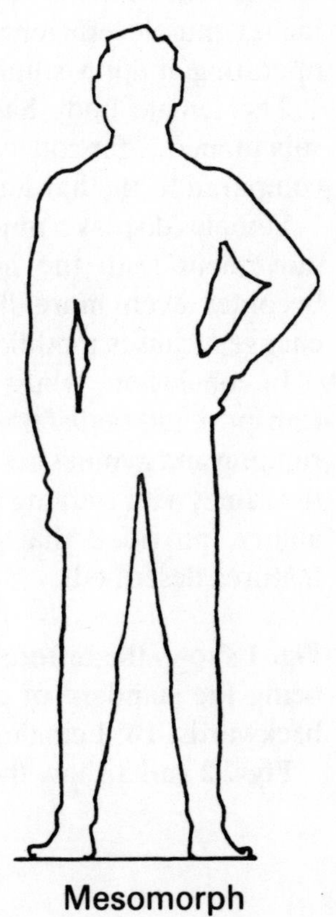

Mesomorph

SIZE AND SEX

Children of both sexes are nearly identical skeletally and muscularly until the growth acceleration of adolescence, which in girls starts at around the age of 10–11 years and in boys around the 12–13 year bracket.

During this growth spurt, the fast-growing new bone, joint and muscle tissue may be susceptible to damage, both in terms of heavy joint and muscle loading and by too many repetitions of the same movements. Care should be taken to vary the training and not impose heavy loads during this transition from child to adult.

In adulthood the muscular and skeletal differences of male and female become significant and are both absolute and in proportion to their height. The average height differential between the sexes is approximately 7 per cent, regardless of race or tribe, the average British heights being 5 ft 10 ins (1,778 mm) and 5 ft 5 ins (1,651 mm) respectively.

Proportionately the female pelvis is deeper, broader and more basin-like and tends to be tilted forwards, causing the small of the back to be more concave in an upright posture.

Due to the proportionately broader hips, the thigh bones of the female slope inwards towards the knee at a steeper angle than those of the male, so that the knee joint loads are modified.

In the male the shoulder girdle and rib cage are proportionately broader and deeper and the levers or bones of both arms and legs are longer than those of the female who, having shorter levers in proportion, can on average develop a higher muscle efficiency at around 65 per cent of maximum than the male operating at approximately 50 per cent of maximum.

The female body has a lower centre of gravity and a thicker covering of subcutaneous fat concealing the muscle development and softening the form, compared to the harder, more angular modelling of the male.

Females display a much higher degree of flexibility and a wider basic range of movement than the male, especially pre-menstrually when the backbone becomes even more flexible; this, combined with associated pelvic girdle changes, causes modifications in posture.

In conclusion, whilst other differences, such as heart rate, oxygen uptake/transport and body fat would be very significant in more athletic sports, such as running and gymnastics, in archery terms male and female can be treated much the same, with training pressures appropriate to their build, state of fitness and ability, provided that due attention is given to the few important special features described.

Fig. 1 shows the difference in proportion between male and female, the pelvis being the standard of comparison. **1a**: Male proportions. Inset: pelvis tilted backwards. **1b**: Female proportions. Inset: pelvis tilted forwards.

Figs. 2 and **3** show the modelling of male and female torsos.

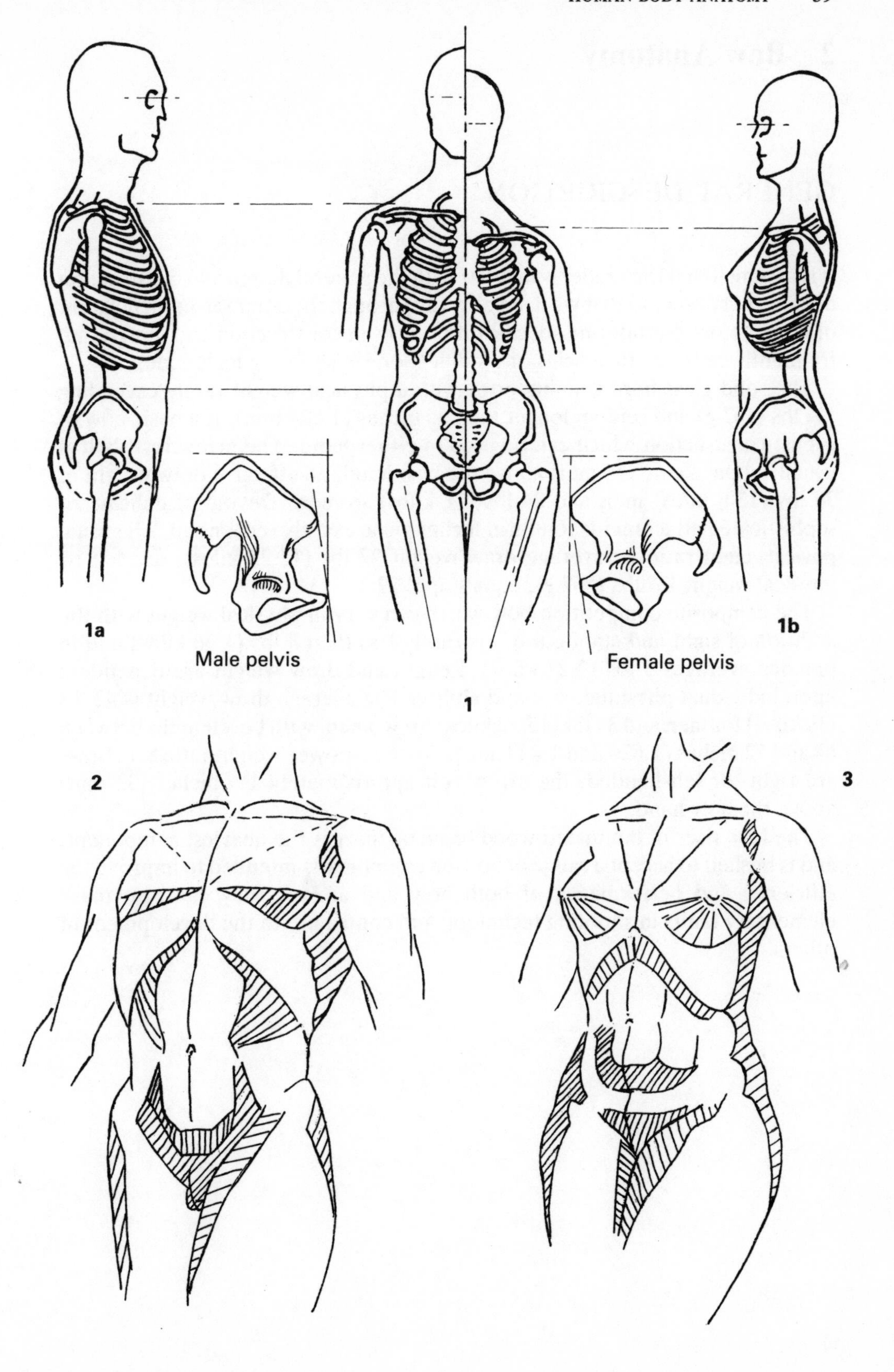
1a
Male pelvis
1
Female pelvis
1b
2
3

2 Bow Anatomy

GENERAL DESCRIPTION

It is assumed that the reader is familiar with the general design and construction of an archery bow, so that we need only run through the common nomenclature of bows before considering specific differences in construction and design that frequently cause inefficiencies or modifications in shooting techniques.

The solid glass fibre training bow, with a physical weight rarely exceeding 1¼ lbs (567 g) and seldom longer than 60 inches (1,524 mm), is a basic bow of robust construction which can be used in either hand. The arrow rest/shelf is usually about ¼ inch (6 mm) above the bow hand, an effective draw weight of 30 lbs (13.6 kilos) men and 24 lbs (11 kilos) women. Devoid of delicate or sophisticated attachments, faults in technique are easily recognised. The usual power/weight ratio is: average draw weight 27 lbs (12.25 kilos), divided by physical weight 1¼ lbs (567 g), equals app. 22:1.

The composite competition bow which can vary in physical weight with the addition of sight and stabilisation, is rarely less than 3 lbs (1.36 kilos) and in practice averages 5 lbs (2.27 kilos). Length and draw weight are dependent upon individual physique, size and ability. The average draw weight is 42 lbs (19 kilos) for men and 34 lbs (15.42 kilos) for women, with bow lengths between 64 and 72 inches (1,626 and 1,829 mm). Average power/weight ratio 8:1. Bows are right- or left-handed, the arrow rest approximately 1¼ inches (32 mm) above the bow hand.

The bow riser of laminated wood or metal alloy is the heaviest component, and is bushed to accept a range of bolt-on components intended to improve the efficiency and performance of both bow and archer; they can also mask elementary faults in shooting technique and contribute to the development of others.

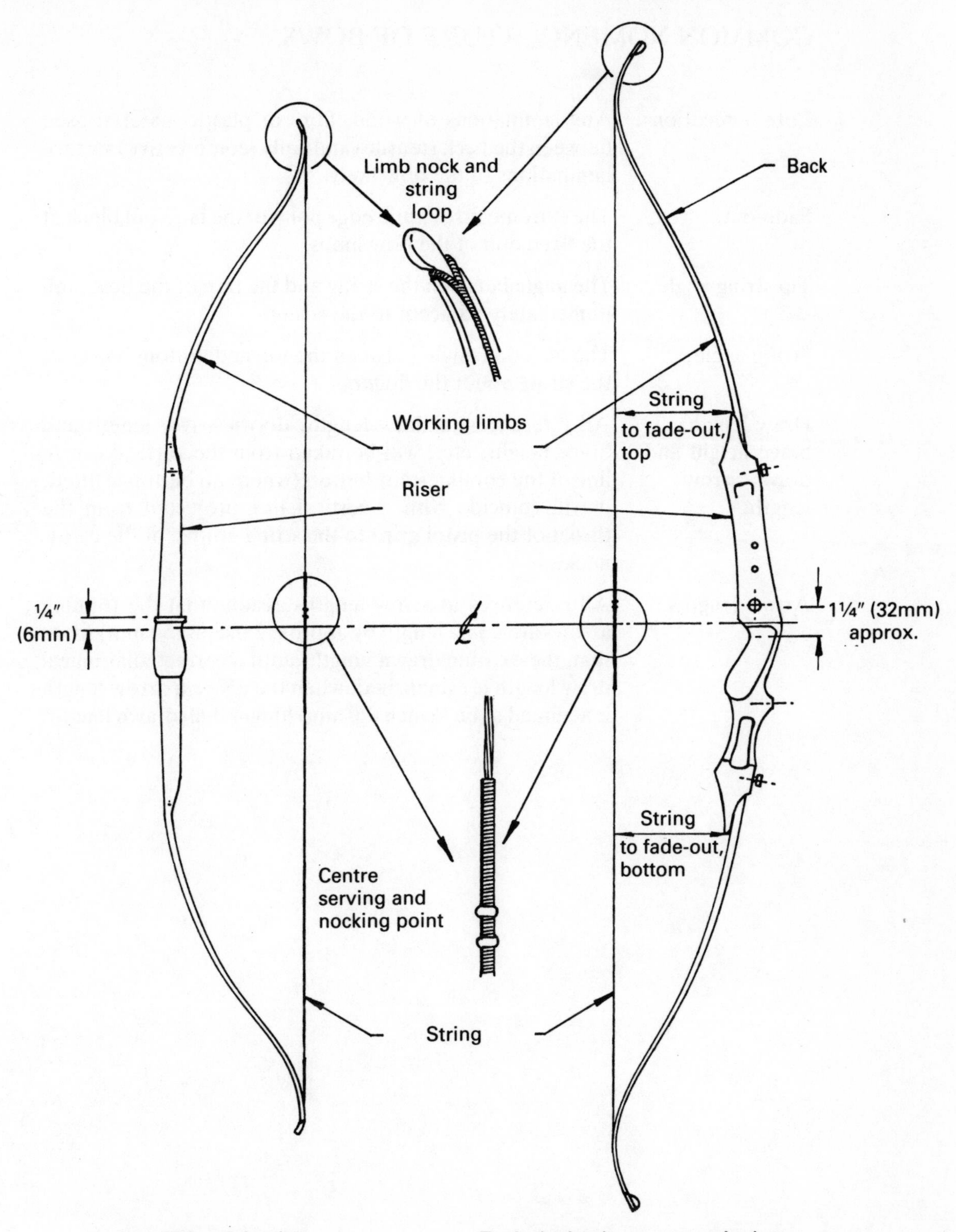

Typical GRP training bow

Typical take-down composite bow

COMMON NOMENCLATURE OF BOWS

Core laminations:	Any laminations of wood, fibre or plastic material used between the back (tensile) and belly (compressive) surface laminations of the bow limbs.
Fade-out:	The extreme tip or knife edge point of the fade-out block at the fixed end of the bow limbs.
Tip string angle:	The angle between the string and the face of the bow limb immediately adjacent to the string.
String angle:	The included angle between the top and bottom halves of the string about the fingers.
Draw length, brace height and drawn arrow length:	All references to draw length, drawn arrow length and brace height, etc., will be taken from the vertical centre line of the compensator button (where no button is fitted, it will coincide with a vertical line projected from the throat of the pistol grip) to the string groove of the arrow nock.
Arrow lengths:	All references to arrow lengths assume that the training arrows are a *safe* length by approx. 2 inches (50 mm) more than the existing drawn length, until a correct anatomical draw length is established, when the *efficient* arrow length is assumed to be ¾ inch (20 mm) longer than drawn length.

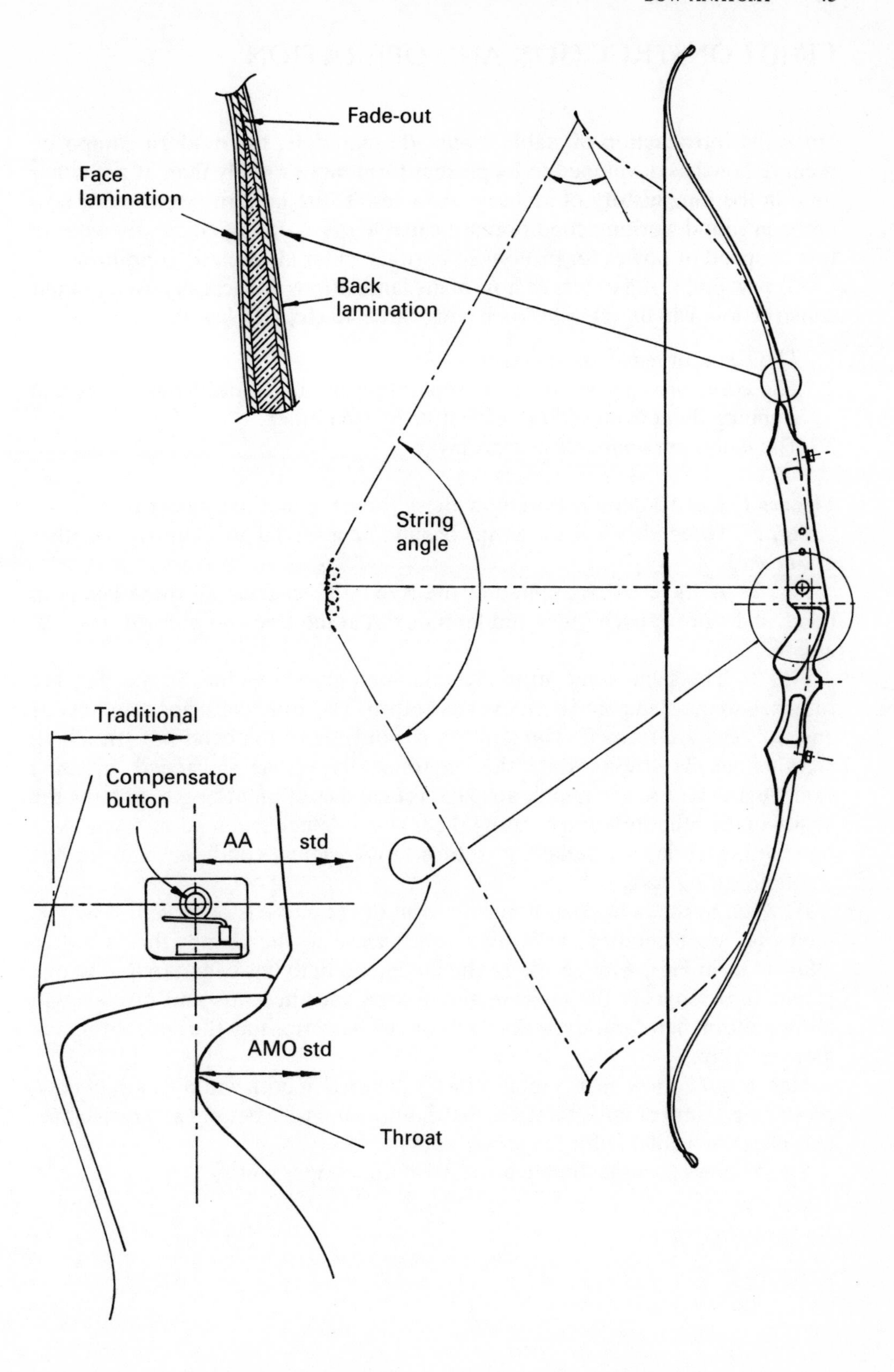
Fade-out
Face lamination
Back lamination
String angle
Traditional
Compensator button
AA
std
AMO std
Throat

LIMB CONSTRUCTION AND OPERATION

Since the introduction of stable manmade materials, the modern composite recurve bow has developed to its present form more rapidly than at any other time in the long history of archery. As a result, the majority of modern bow limbs in sound working condition are capable of operating efficiently without loss of speed or power for prolonged periods under all climatic conditions.

All bow limbs, regardless of how many laminations are actually used in their construction, can be regarded as having three mechanical layers.

1 The back, or *tensile stress* layer.
2 The core, or *sheer stress* layer, separating the back and front layers and stopping them from sliding respective to each other.
3 The belly, or *compressive stress* layer.

Figures 1, **2** and **3** demonstrate how these three stresses are created.

Fig. 1 Three identical-size strips of suitable material are clamped together at one end.

Fig. 2 A force 'A' is applied at the free ends, causing all three layers to bend, sliding over each other and fanning out at the free end to form steps 'B' and 'C'.

Fig. 3 The same three strips, having been glued together in the flat, are returned to the clamp and bent over as before. This time the strips cannot slide and no steps are formed. The strip on the outside of the bend has stretched, creating tensile stress, while the innermost layer has shortened, creating compressive stress. The middle strip has retained its original length, fighting the action of the other two and creating sheer stress. When the bending force 'A' is removed, each layer attempts to return to its original condition, causing the whole to spring back.

If, when in the bent condition, the form of the curve is observed, it will be seen that most bending, or stress, occurs close to the clamp; this is not as efficient as in **Figs. 4** and **5** where the laminated limb has been tapered in one plane, thus reducing the cross-sectional area and the mass and producing a more uniform bend and stress distribution, while permitting the limb to recover more quickly.

Figs. 6 and **7** show an assembly which is tapered in both width and thickness, producing a limb of uniform stress distribution and with better twist resistance, and material available for the string nock.

Fig. 8 shows a simple limb construction for comparison.

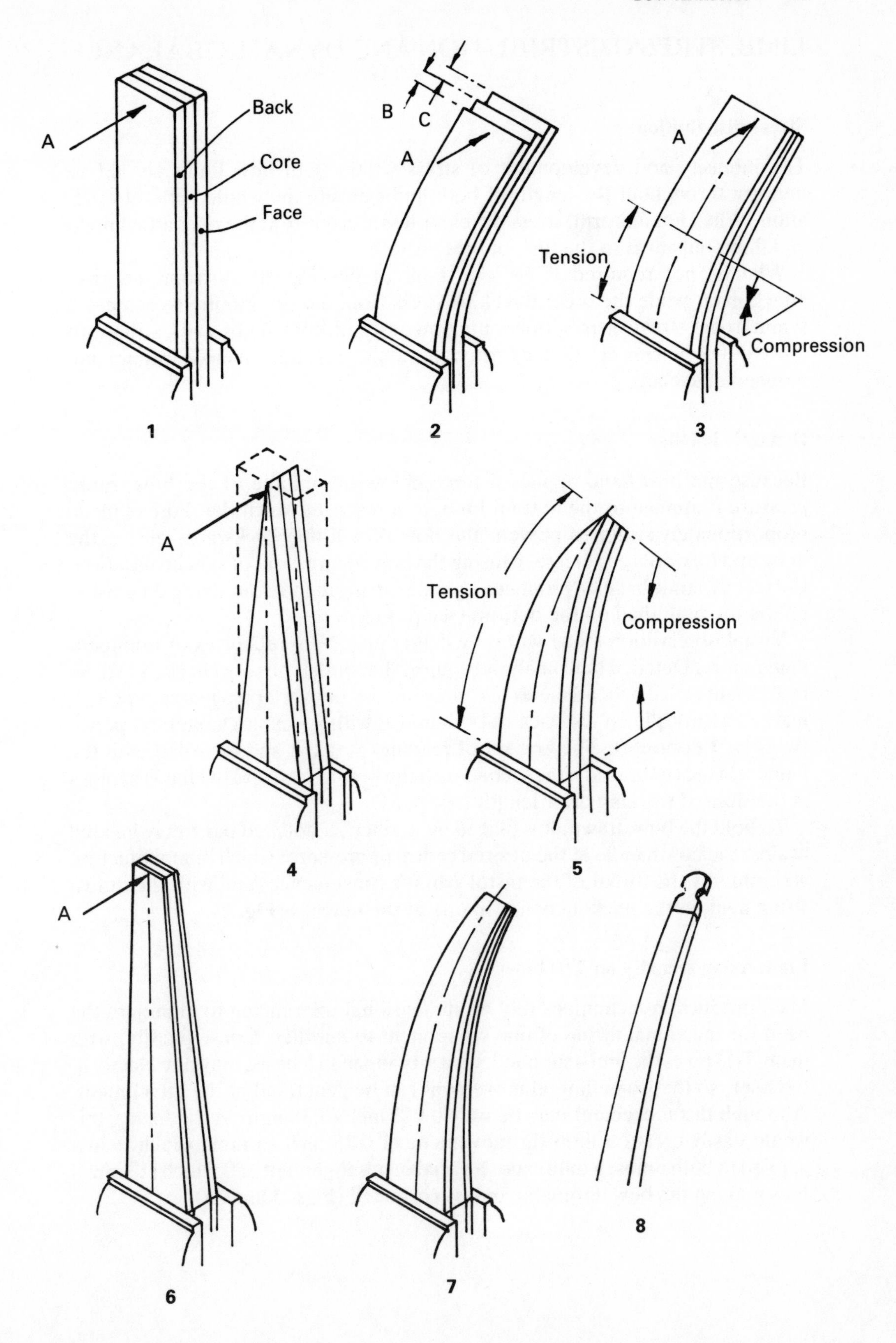
A
Back
Core
Face
1
B
C
A
2
A
Tension
Compression
3
A
4
Tension
Compression
5
A
6
7
8

LIMB. STRESS DISTRIBUTION AND DYNAMIC BALANCE

Stress distribution

The intensity and development of stress within both bow limbs should be uniform throughout the length of both limbs during the whole cycle of operation. When not uniform, stress develops less efficiently at the riser attachment and flows outwards to the tips, or vice versa.

What is not required is for one limb to develop stress from the riser attachment, while the other develops stress from the tip. Failure to achieve a symmetrical stress distribution simultaneously in both limbs causes them to move out of synchronisation, a form of instability resulting in inconsistency and reduced efficiency.

Dynamic balance

Because the bow hand applies a force below the middle of the bow, more pressure is applied to the bottom limb, as a result of which that limb is made proportionately stiffer to prevent the bow riser tilting backwards during the draw and forwards on release, causing the bow to move out of synchronisation. Correct dynamic balance produces a greater string to fade-out/fixing dimension on the top limb than on the bottom (see p. 41).

Visual observation alone will only detect major discrepancies or imminent limb failure. Detailed limb analysis requires that both limbs are checked with an instrument called a 'bend meter' or 'circle meter' at overlapping station points, marked identically on the back of both limbs, with a wax or chinagraph pencil (see **Fig. 1** opposite). The first set of readings is taken and recorded with the limbs relaxed (unbraced), the second with the bow braced and the final readings at the desired working draw length (see p. 51).

To hold the bow drawn, it is placed on a 'tiller', a notched bar freely located against the bow handle at the desired centre of pressure, which in manufacture is commonly the throat of the pistol grip for convenience, and with the drawn string held, at the nocking point, in one of the notches (**Fig. 2**).

Limb fixing security on T/D bows

Mass production techniques rely on dimensional tolerancing to eliminate the need for individual fitting of one component to another. Consequently, with many T/D bows the limbs supplied, on a mix and match basis, may not exactly fit the riser, so that some lateral movement can be generated at the attachment. Although this movement may be only 0.015 inch (0.38 mm) at the fixing, this would easily create a limb tip movement of 0.25 inch (6 mm) which, when applied to both limbs, would cause a variable misalignment of 0.5 inch (13 mm), thus making the bow untunable unless corrected (**Figs. 3** and **3a**).

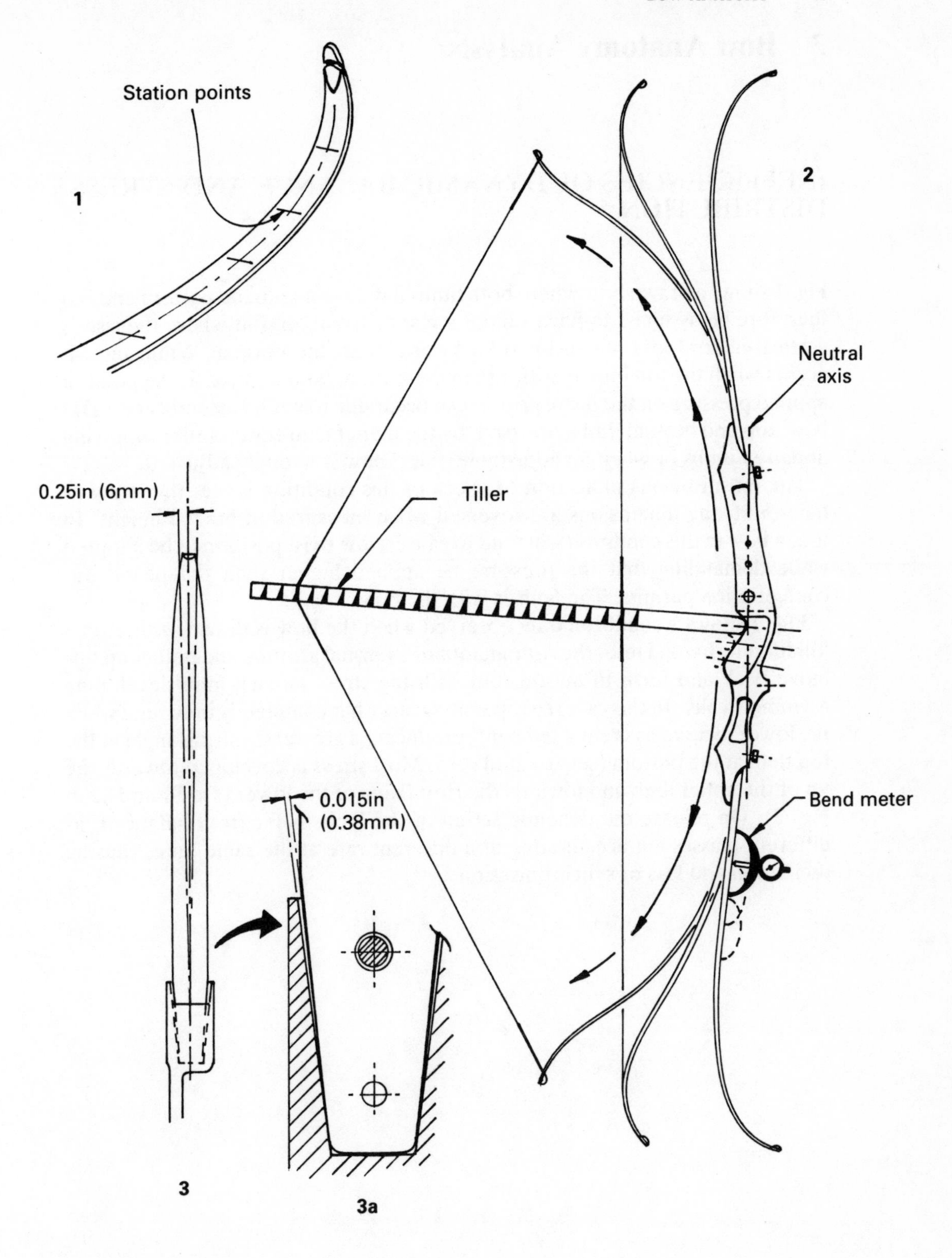
Station points
1
2
Neutral axis
0.25in (6mm)
Tiller
Bend meter
0.015in (0.38mm)
3
3a

3 Bow Anatomy Analysis

INEFFICIENCIES OF DYNAMIC BALANCE AND STRESS DISTRIBUTION

Fig. 1 shows a drawn bow where both limbs have a similar bend pattern and can therefore be assumed to have similar stress distribution, but where the riser's vertical neutral axis has inclined backwards from the normal. While rare, it occurs when the top limb is stiffer than the bottom limb relative to the point of applied pressure on the pistol grip. It can occur due to wrong assembly of a T/D bow, top and bottom limbs reversed, by the manufacturer or retailer supplying unpaired limbs or when an adjustable 'tiller' bow is wrongly adjusted.

The most obvious indication or check of this condition is that the string to fade-out/fixing dimensions are reversed when measured at braced height. In use, a bow in this condition will tend to cause a low wrist position to be adopted while demanding that the pressure be applied higher than the pistol grip configuration permits. The fault is with the bow.

Fig. 2 shows a condition only observed when the bow is drawn, either on a 'tiller' or by hand. Here, the riser maintains a normal attitude and both limp tips move back and forth in unison, but with the stress in each limb developing asymmetrically. In this case the top limb recurve has completely unwound while the lower recurve has remained bent, producing a greater tip string angle at the top than at the bottom (see $\theta+$ and $\theta-$). Most stress is developed towards the tip of the upper limb and towards the riser fixing of the lower (see S1 and S2 in Fig. 2). On release the dynamic action of the limbs is far from balanced, as different masses are accelerating at a different rate at the same time, causing oscillation and loss of synchronisation.

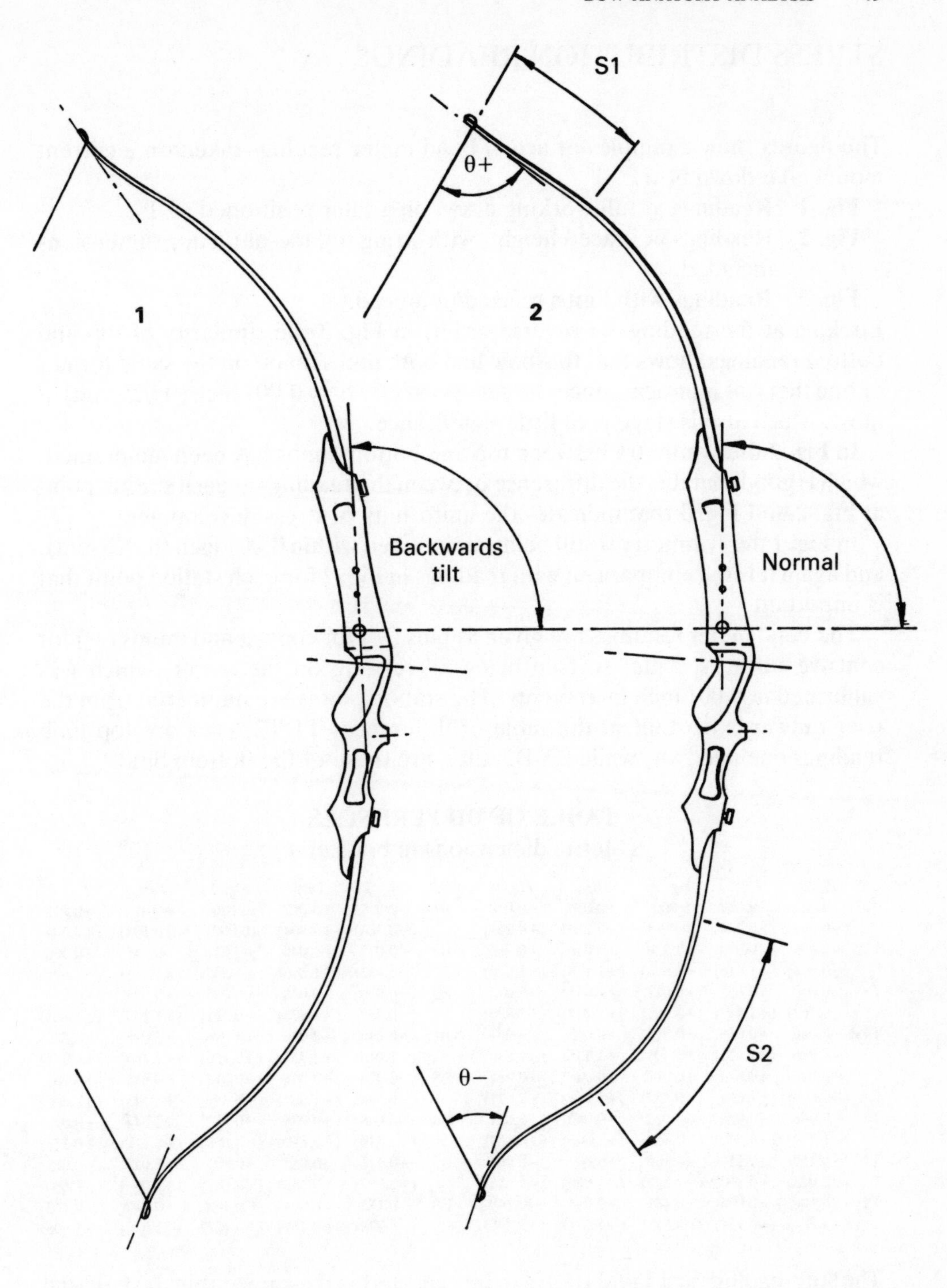
S1
θ+
1
2
Backwards
tilt
Normal
S2
θ−

STRESS DISTRIBUTION READINGS

The figures show examples of actual bend meter readings taken on a current model take-down bow:

Fig. 1 Readings at full working draw, on a tiller positioned at 'P'.
Fig. 2 Readings at braced height, with string to fade-out/fixing dimensions included.
Fig. 3 Readings with limbs relaxed/unbraced.

Looking at the readings in reverse order, in **Fig. 3** the similarity of top and bottom readings shows that this bow had both limbs made on the same former or one that was identical, since the curves vary by only 0.001 inch (0.025 mm) at most, which at this stage is of little significance.

In **Fig. 2** the symmetry between top and bottom limbs has been maintained, which is good, but it is the difference between the readings at each station point at Fig. 2 and Fig. 3 that indicates the uniformity of stress development.

In **Fig. 1** the symmetry is still being maintained within 0.001 inch (0.025 mm), and again it is the comparison with readings in Fig. 2 for each station point that is important.

The bend meter readings are given as plus (+) for convex and minus (−) for concave surfaces, a flat surface being '0' reading on the meter, which was calibrated in 0.001 inch increments. The station points are numbered from the riser outwards, so that in the table of differences T1 T2, etc., are top limb readings one and two, while B1 B2, etc., are those of the bottom limb.

TABLE OF DIFFERENCES
(Metric dimensions in brackets)

S/P	*Fig. 3*	*Diff.*	*Fig. 2*	*Diff.*	*Fig. 1*	*S/P*	*Fig. 3*	*Diff.*	*Fig. 2*	*Diff.*	*Fig. 1*
T1	−0.012	+0.012	0.000	+0.010	+0.010	B1	−0.012	+0.012	0.000	+0.012	+0.012
	(−0.304)	(+0.304)	(0.000)	(+0.254)	(+0.254)		(−0.304)	(+0.304)	(0.000)	(+0.304)	(+0.304)
T2	−0.020	+0.040	+0.020	+0.046	+0.066	B2	−0.019	+0.040	+0.021	+0.045	+0.066
	(−0.508)	(+1.016)	(+0.508)	(+1.168)	(+1.676)		(−0.482)	(+1.016)	(+0.533)	(+1.143)	(+1.676)
T3	−0.030	+0.057	+0.027	+0.045	+0.072	B3	−0.030	+0.058	+0.028	+0.045	+0.073
	(−0.762)	(+1.447)	(+0.685)	(+1.143)	(+1.828)		(−0.762)	(+1.473)	(+0.711)	(+1.143)	(+1.854)
T4	−0.040	+0.056	+0.016	+0.045	+0.061	B4	−0.040	+0.056	+0.016	*+0.046**	+0.062
	(−1.016)	(+1.422)	(+0.406)	(+1.143)	(+1.549)		(−1.016)	(+1.422)	(+0.406)	*(+1.168)*	(+1.574)
T5	−0.024	+0.042	+0.018	*+0.046**	+0.064	B5	−0.023	+0.041	+0.018	+0.045	+0.063
	(−0.609)	(+1.066)	(+0.457)	*(+1.168)*	(+1.625)		(−0.584)	(+1.041)	(+0.457)	(+1.143)	(+1.600)
T6	−0.048	+0.026	−0.022	+0.043	+0.021	B6	−0.048	+0.026	−0.022	+0.044	+0.022
	(−1.219)	(+0.660)	(−0.558)	(+1.092)	(+0.533)		(−1.219)	(+0.660)	(−0.558)	(+1.117)	(+0.558)
T7	−0.119	+0.013	−0.106	+0.042	−0.064	B7	−0.118	+0.013	−0.105	+0.042	−0.063
	(−3.022)	(+0.330)	(−2.692)	(+1.066)	(−1.625)		(−2.997)	(+0.330)	(−2.667)	(+1.066)	(−1.600)
T8	−0.186	+0.005	−0.181	+0.041	−0.140	B8	−0.186	+0.004	−0.182	+0.040	−0.142
	(−4.724)	(+0.127)	(−4.597)	(+1.041)	(−3.556)		(−4.724)	(+0.101)	(−4.622)	(+1.016)	(−3.606)

The stiff readings at T1 and B1 are to be expected as they are within the fade-out block; if one had shown a significant difference there would be cause for concern.

A slight weakness exists at T5* and B4*, but being only 0.001 inch (0.025 mm) out of step could be attributed to the meter being calibrated by the same increment. It is therefore insignificant; a difference of 0.003 inch (0.076 mm) or greater, would be cause for consideration.

The working recurves could be improved since T7, T8, B7 and B8 show this area to the stiff, although the improvement in recovery speed may not be of significance except to an elite performer.

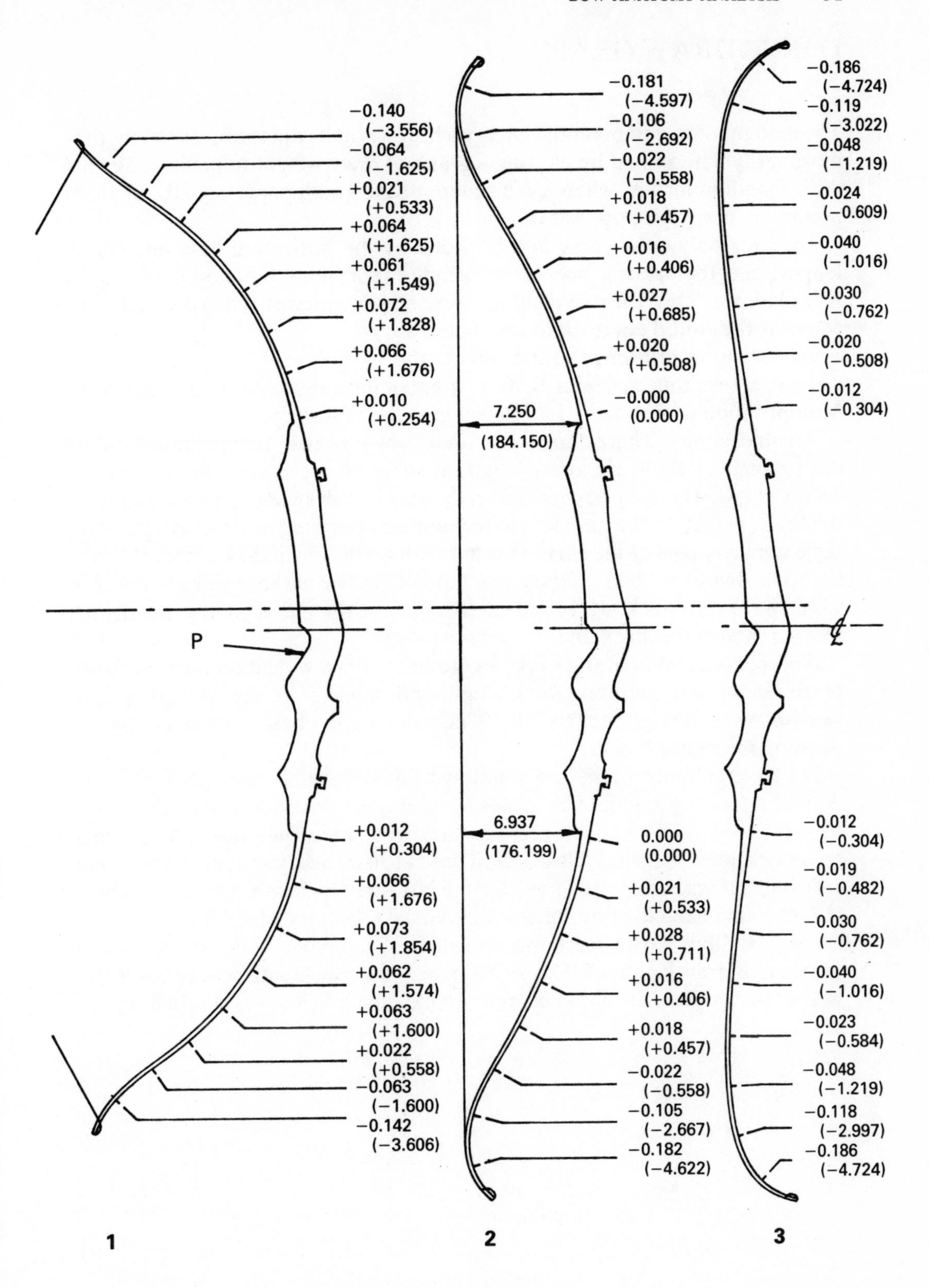

−0.140
(−3.556)
−0.064
(−1.625)
+0.021
(+0.533)
+0.064
(+1.625)
+0.061
(+1.549)
+0.072
(+1.828)
+0.066
(+1.676)
+0.010
(+0.254)
P
+0.012
(+0.304)
+0.066
(+1.676)
+0.073
(+1.854)
+0.062
(+1.574)
+0.063
(+1.600)
+0.022
(+0.558)
−0.063
(−1.600)
−0.142
(−3.606)
1
−0.181
(−4.597)
−0.106
(−2.692)
−0.022
(−0.558)
+0.018
(+0.457)
+0.016
(+0.406)
+0.027
(+0.685)
+0.020
(+0.508)
−0.000
(0.000)
7.250
(184.150)
6.937
(176.199)
0.000
(0.000)
+0.021
(+0.533)
+0.028
(+0.711)
+0.016
(+0.406)
+0.018
(+0.457)
−0.022
(−0.558)
−0.105
(−2.667)
−0.182
(−4.622)
2
−0.186
(−4.724)
−0.119
(−3.022)
−0.048
(−1.219)
−0.024
(−0.609)
−0.040
(−1.016)
−0.030
(−0.762)
−0.020
(−0.508)
−0.012
(−0.304)
−0.012
(−0.304)
−0.019
(−0.482)
−0.030
(−0.762)
−0.040
(−1.016)
−0.023
(−0.584)
−0.048
(−1.219)
−0.118
(−2.997)
−0.186
(−4.724)
3

FORCE/DRAW GRAPH

The amount of stored potential energy a bow has at its operating draw length is most easily determined by plotting a graph of draw weight in pounds, against draw length in inches, where each square of the graph paper equals one inch/pound of energy (see opposite).

The area below the curve and bounded by the horizontal base line (draw length) and the vertical line (draw weight) represents the stored energy in pound/inches. This, the sum of all squares and part squares, when divided by 12 converts the stored energy into foot/pounds.

To obtain an efficiency rating, divide the foot/pounds by operating draw weight: a resulting figure of 0.90 or greater indicates a very efficient bow. Multiplication of this figure by 100 will give the efficiency.

An undesirable characteristic of some bows is that the poundage soars disproportionately to the draw length at some point, a condition commonly called 'stack'. This may be checked on the graph by drawing a straight line from the brace height on the base line to the desired operating draw length point on the curve; any part of the curve that falls below this line indicates that the bow has some degree of stack. If the curve follows the line without going below it, it would have zero stack, while one that is all above the line is good to the degree that it is above the stack line.

Another indication of stack is to ascertain the draw weight mid-way between brace height and operating draw length and divide it by the operating draw weight. Any figure greater than 0.55 indicates a good bow, with larger figures showing the better bows.

For the graph shown, the bow was drawn and weighed to one inch beyond the desired operating length of 29 inches to ascertain when stack occurred. As can be seen, used at 29 inches this bow is stack free, and would not be worse than zero stack at 29.50 inches. However, if used at 30 inches, a new stack line would indicate that stacking would exist for the last three inches of operation, just at the most undesirable point for the anatomical efficiency of the archer.

As it is, this particular bow is ideal for an archer with an established anatomical draw length of 29 to 29.50 inches, since at this draw length not only has no stack occurred, but maximum usable bow efficiency is reached.

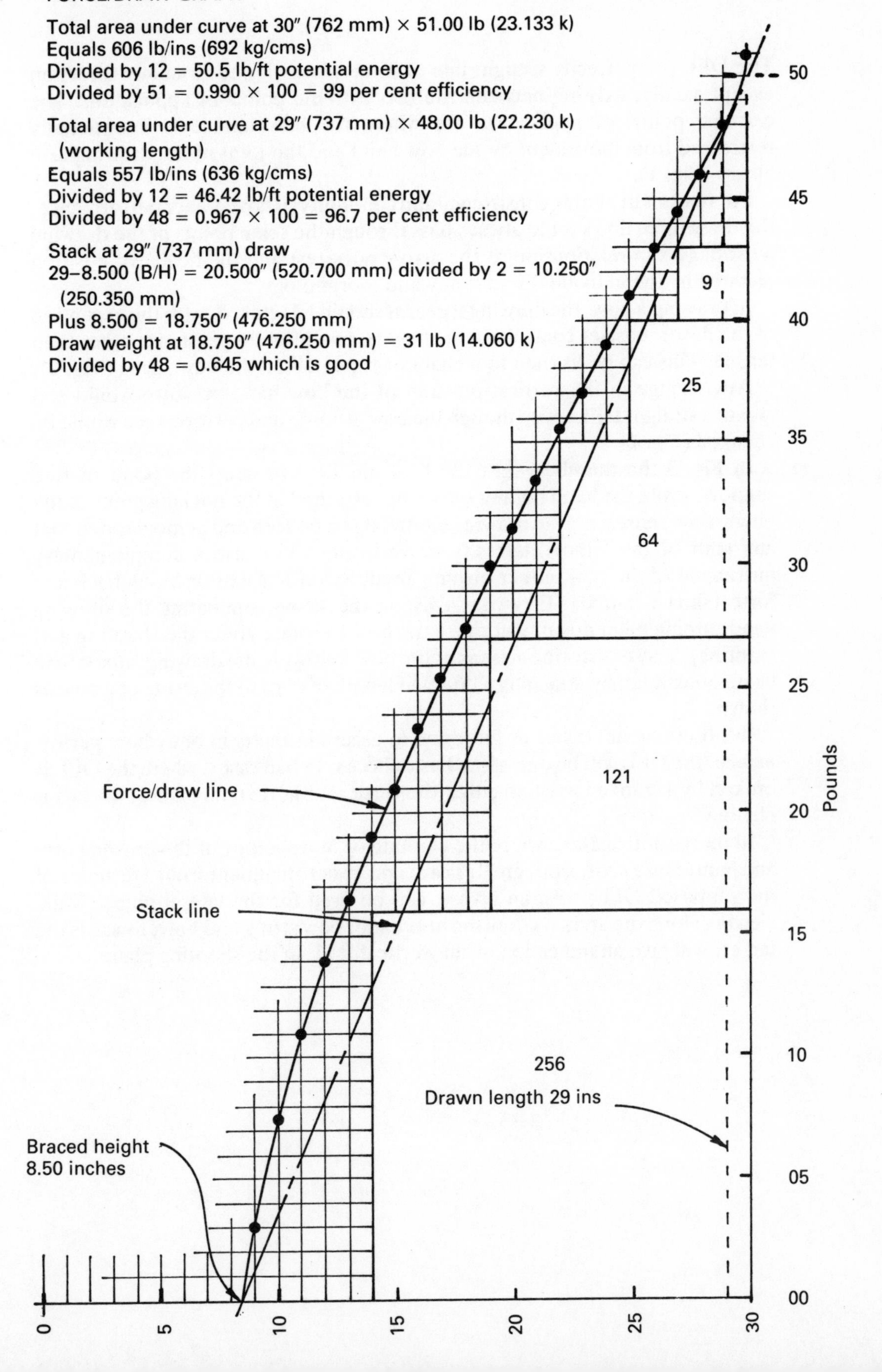

FORCE/DRAW GRAPH
Total area under curve at 30″ (762 mm) × 51.00 lb (23.133 k)
Equals 606 lb/ins (692 kg/cms)
Divided by 12 = 50.5 lb/ft potential energy
Divided by 51 = 0.990 × 100 = 99 per cent efficiency
Total area under curve at 29″ (737 mm) × 48.00 lb (22.230 k)
(working length)
Equals 557 lb/ins (636 kg/cms)
Divided by 12 = 46.42 lb/ft potential energy
Divided by 48 = 0.967 × 100 = 96.7 per cent efficiency
Stack at 29″ (737 mm) draw
29–8.500 (B/H) = 20.500″ (520.700 mm) divided by 2 = 10.250″
(250.350 mm)
Plus 8.500 = 18.750″ (476.250 mm)
Draw weight at 18.750″ (476.250 mm) = 31 lb (14.060 k)
Divided by 48 = 0.645 which is good
Force/draw line
Stack line
Braced height
8.50 inches
Drawn length 29 ins
9
25
64
121
256
Pounds
00
05
10
15
20
25
30
35
40
45
50
0
5
10
15
20
25
30

DRAW FORCE LINE

The DFL is a perfectly straight line of force when viewed from any direction except axially, existing between the two extreme points of application. The extreme points of application are where the bow handle is intentionally restrained from movement by the bow hand and the joint of the drawing arm elbow (**Fig. 1**).

For reasons of aiming consistency and continuity of bow/archer performance, the draw force line should always pass through the same points of the drawing wrist/fingers in relationship to the arrow nock/rest and the head/eye position dictated by the individual's anatomy and morphology.

In drawing a bow, the drawing forearm should be relaxed, with the exception of the flexor muscles controlling the fingers, and offer no resistance other than tensile. This can be likened to a chain or rope pulling the bow string (**Fig. 2**).

Any change in the vertical position of the bow hand pressure would still create a straight DFL, even though the bow attitude and performance would be changed (**Fig. 2**).

In **Fig. 3** the thumb against the bow handle represents the point of free support, while the hand pulling the string, attached at the nocking point of the bow string, represents the drawing elbow. It can be seen and demonstrated that any shift of the 'elbow' laterally or vertically will cause a complementary movement of the bow, either turning about its vertical axis or tilting back and forth (shown dotted). Likewise, twisting the string, simulating the drawing hand turning palm down, will cause the bow to rotate about the shooting axis (canting). These castoring actions of the bow following the drawing 'elbow' can be demonstrated by attaching a doubled length of cord to the string of a bow as shown.

In observing an archer at full draw to ascertain faults in body/bow performance, the DFL will be one of the basic checks. In bad cases, where the DFL is broken by a cranked wrist, in either the vertical or horizontal planes, the fact is obvious.

In more subtle cases, where the clothing or morphology of the drawing arm and hand cause confusion, greater care and visual alignment from a distance of the supposed DFL, with an arrow, can be used for the lateral plane, while viewing along the archer's drawing arm/hand, bow string and bow, towards the target, will give an indication of the vertical DFL in the shooting plane.

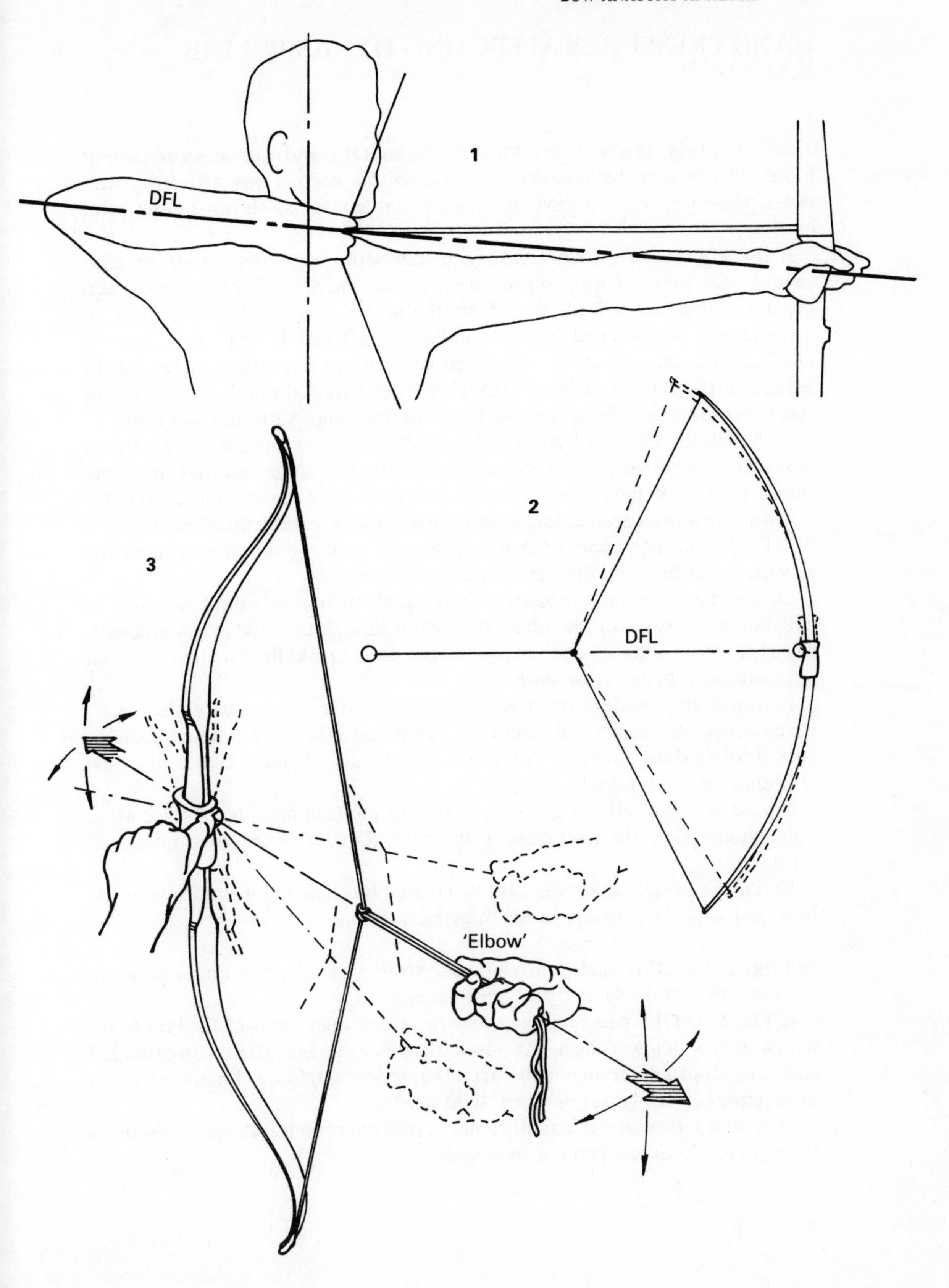
1
DFL
2
DFL
3
'Elbow'

HAND PRESSURES AFFECTING DYNAMIC LIMB BALANCE

This archer (**Fig. 1**) always develops an efficient DFL and produces a consistent loose. The bow is dynamically balanced for his normal bow hand pressure point, shown as 'N', the bow adopting a stable state as shown by the solid outline.

If for any reason—a new pistol grip, deliberate experimentation or pure chance—the point of applied pressure is raised and a new DFL created, then the top of the riser will tilt away from the archer, causing the upper limb to become more stressed and the lower limb stress reduced. If the pressure point is lowered, the top limb stress is reduced and bottom limb stress increased. In either case the dynamic balance of the bow is destroyed, the limbs moving out of synchronisation on release and the arrow performance suffering as a result.

Although the effects of non-synchronisation may be seen, if severe, by an observer or felt in the hand by the archer, they frequently get ignored due to the change in the sight pin height relative to the arrow angle of elevation, as follows:

With a forwards extended sight, as shown in **Fig. 1**, raising the pressure point to 'H' tilts the riser and sight forwards with little or no change to arrow elevation, but bringing the sight pin effectively lower.

On coming to the aim the bow is raised slightly higher, elevating the arrow to a higher trajectory with the effect that, even though the bow is less efficient, since the arrow is higher on the target at the short to middle distances it is seen as producing a better sight mark.

Lowering the pressure point to 'L' would, with a forward extended sight, have the opposite effect and would be abandoned as giving worse sight marks, even if with a different bow, with a different dynamic balance centre, the bow efficiency were improved.

Similar opposite effects are produced with inboard mounted sights, while sights mounted on the riser close to the neutral axis give the least noticeable error.

Variations in sight mark can also be created by changing the attitude of the bow riser with the pressure of the drawing fingers.

In (**Fig. 1**) the DFL passes through the arrow nock, the first finger pressure equalling that of the second and third fingers.

In **Fig. 2** the DFL passes either above the arrow nock, causing the bow to tilt backwards, or below, causing the bow to tilt forwards. In each case an extended sight will adopt a different alignment and cause a new arrow inclination to give a false impression of better or worse sight marks.

One clear indication of lost efficiency is that over the full range of distances the sight marks expand on the sight scale.

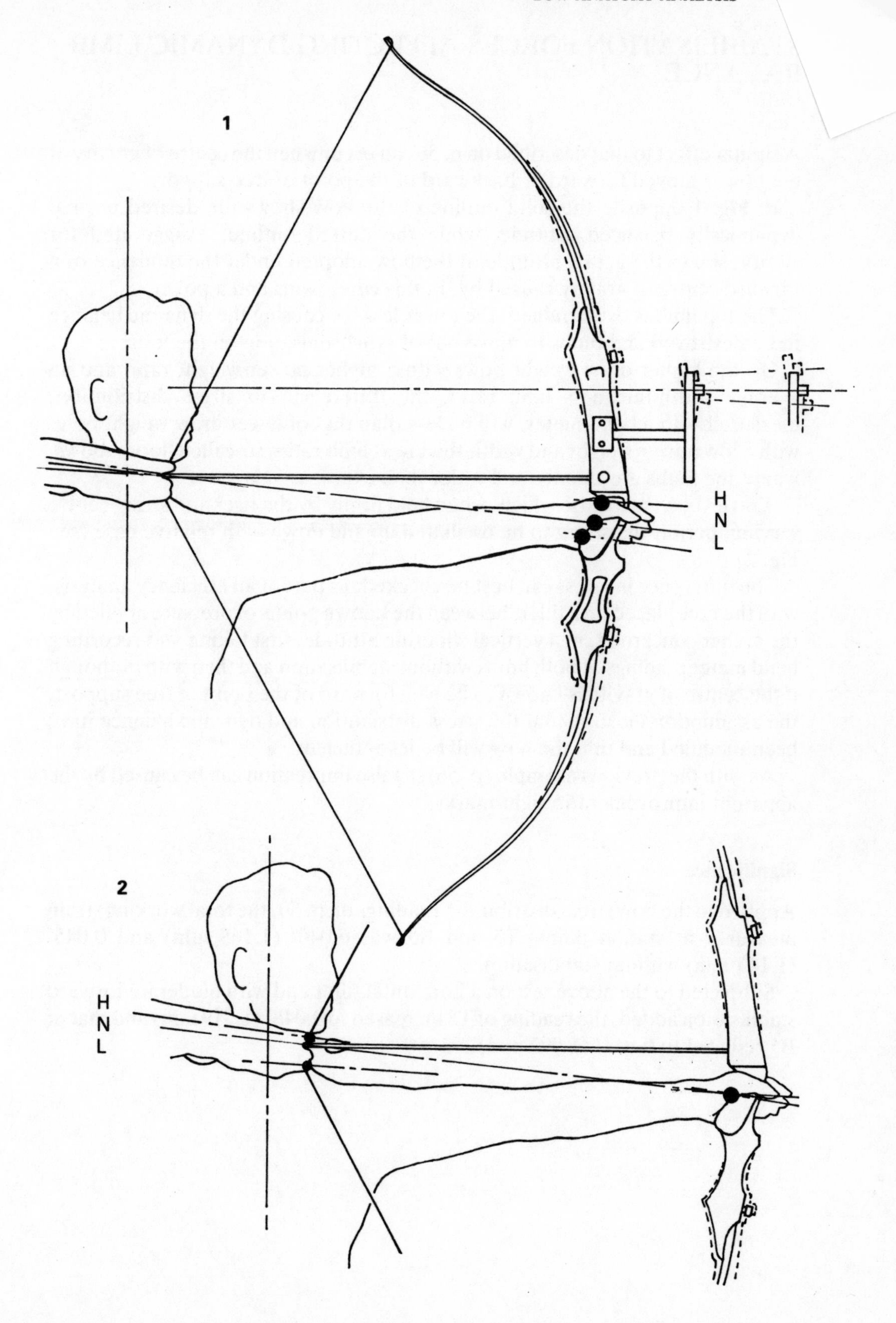
1
H
N
L
2
H
N
L

STABILISATION FORCES AFFECTING DYNAMIC LIMB BALANCE

A similar effect to that described on p. 56 can occur when the centre of gravity of the bow is moved forward or backward of the point of free support.

In **Fig. 1** opposite the solid outline of the bow shows the desired normal dynamically balanced attitude, while the dotted outline, exaggerated for clarity, shows the actual attitude of the bow adopted under the influence of a forward centre of gravity caused by, in this case, twins and a poker.

The top limb is overstrained, the lower less so, causing the dynamic balance to be destroyed and limbs to move out of synchronisation on the loose.

On the higher draw weight bows with a higher power/weight ratio and an average width/thickness limb ratio, the differences in stress distribution, measured with a bend meter, will be less than that of lower draw weight bows with a low power/weight and width/thickness limb ratio, so-called 'loose' bows, where the limbs are thinner and wider than average.

'Loose' bows are those which, when held firmly by the riser and string centre serving, permit the string to be oscillated up and down with relative ease (see **Fig. 2**).

The difference in stress can best be checked, as part of an efficiency analysis, with the bow placed on a tiller, between the known points of pressure applied by the archer concerned, in a vertical shooting attitude, first taking and recording bend meter readings of both limbs without stabilisation and then with, although if the centre of gravity is known to be well forward of the point of free support, the assumption must be that the stress distribution and dynamic balance have been modified and that the bow will be less efficient.

As with the previous example (p. 56), a false impression can be caused by the apparent improvement in sight marks.

Significance

Applied to the bow stress distribution readings on p. 50, the total working strain measured at station points T5 and B5 was 0.046″ (1.168 mm) and 0.045″ (1.143 mm) without stabilisation.

Subjected to the above test on a horizontal tiller and with moderate forward stabilisation added, the reading of T5 increased to 0.048″ (1.219 mm) and that of B5 reduced to 0.043″ (1.092 mm).

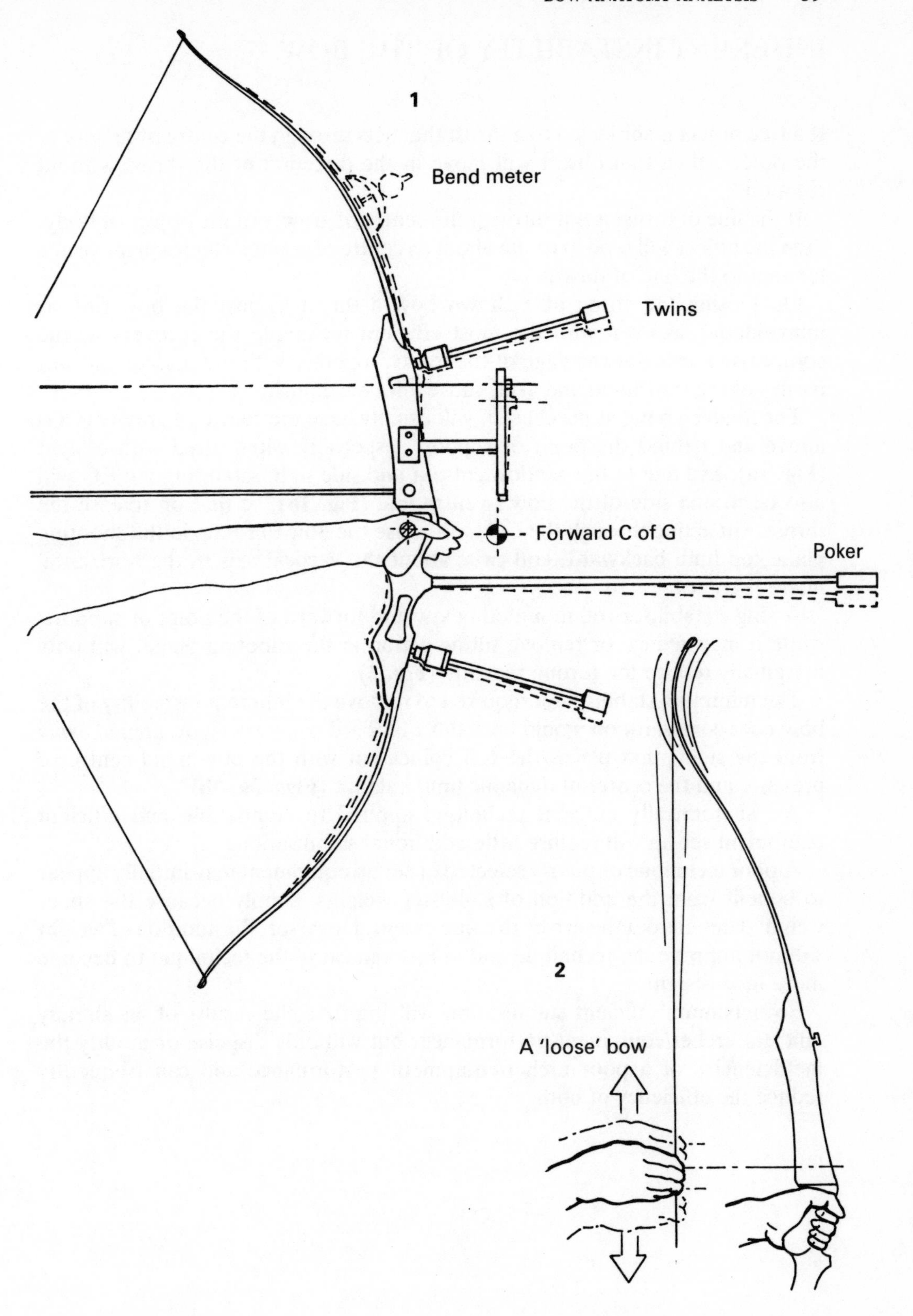
1
Bend meter
Twins
Forward C of G
Poker
2
A 'loose' bow

INHERENT INSTABILITY OF THE BOW

If a free object is subjected to a thrust that acts through the centre of gravity of the object, then that object will move in the direction of the thrust without rotation.

If the line of thrust is not through the centre of gravity of the object or body, then the object will tend to rotate about its centre of gravity which will move at a tangent to the line of thrust.

On loosing the string of a drawn bow a thrust against the bow riser is unavoidable, as even with the most efficient technique the recovery of the compressed articular cartilage of the joints, together with the muscle and soft tissues of the bow hand and arm, cause a forward push.

The modern bow, as purchased, will usually have the centre of gravity (CG) above and behind the point of support, especially when fitted with a sight (**Fig. 1a**), and due to the window cut-out and side sight mounting the CG will also be to one side of the bow's centre line (**Fig. 1b**), so that on release the thrust, not acting through the CG, will cause the bow to rotate in the shooting plane top limb backward, and twist about the vertical axis in the horizontal plane (**Fig. 1c**).

A single stabiliser rod mounted below and forward of the point of support, while it may reduce or remove tilting action in the shooting plane, will only marginally reduce the torque reaction (**Fig. 2**).

The minimum stabilisation required to remove the inherent instability of the bow riser configuration would be a short inboard counterweight, angled away from the sight, that places the CG coincident with the bow hand centre of pressure and the centre of dynamic limb balance (**Figs. 3a**, **3b**).

An anatomically efficient technique applied to compatible and efficient equipment set-up will require little additional stabilisation.

A poor technique or poorly selected or set up equipment may initially appear to benefit from the addition of stabiliser weights, simply because the sheer weight dampens out the errors to some extent. However, the addition of weight will not improve the technique and in fact can cause the technique to become more inconsistent.

So maximum efficient stabilisation will improve the results of an already efficient archer/equipment performance, but will only disguise or modify the inefficiencies of a poor archer/equipment performance and can frequently reduce the efficiency of both.

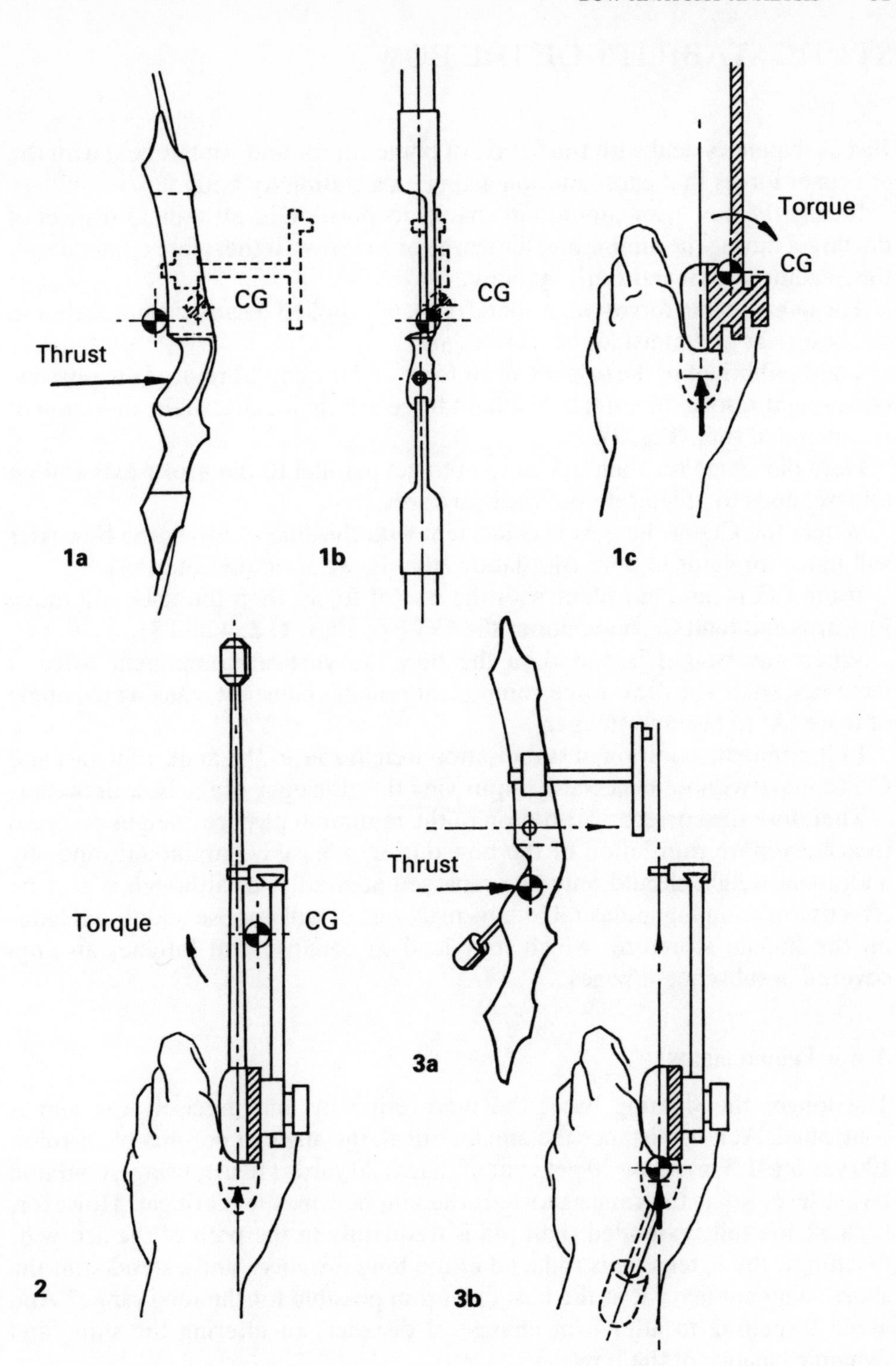
CG
Thrust
1a
CG
1b
Torque
CG
1c
Torque
CG
2
Thrust
3a
3b

STATIC STABILITY OF THE BOW

Just as dynamics deal with the action of bodies in motion, statics deal with the effects of forces that cause motion acting on a stationary body.

Ideally the bow riser should not change its position or attitude in respect of the target during the aiming and discharge of an arrow; it therefore comes under the heading statics and static stability.

The unavoidable forces, mentioned on p. 60, applied by an efficient archer to the bow riser at the instant of release, are:

The equilibriant of the original draw force and the equilibriant of the physical bow weight resolve to a single resultant force acting, ideally, in the direction of the intended shot (**Fig. 3**).

Here the single resultant 'A' is seen to act parallel to the arrow axis and on release tends to accelerate the riser forwards.

Where the CG of the bow is coincident with this line of force, the bow riser will move forwards in pure translation (that is, without any rotation).

If the CG is not coincident with the line of force, then the riser will move forwards and tend to rotate about the CG (see **Figs. 1**, **2**, **4** and **5**).

When any weight is added to the bow the vertical component force is increased while the draw force component remains constant, causing the angle of force 'A' to become steeper.

Indiscriminate addition of stabilisation weight causes the angle of thrust and CG to move without necessarily improving the efficiency of the bow or archer.

Therefore the correct distribution of the minimum physical weight practical to achieve pure translation of the bow during release is paramount, and any additional weight should only be employed advisedly, as although it may be effective in damping undesirable bow reactions, it will impose additional loads on the human structure, which may lead to collapse and fatigue, an area covered in subsequent pages.

A word about sights

The longer the sighting base, the more critically and precisely the aim is controlled. At long distance the aim is critical, the angle of permissible error at 100 yards (91.5 m) being 20 per cent of that at 20 yards (18 m), using a common target face. So as the range shortens the aim becomes less critical. However, because the fully extended sight pin is frequently in the path of the arrow or fletchings, the extension is reduced at the long distances and extended at the short. Why not leave it at the best extension possible for the long range? And avoid forgetting to alter it at change of distance, or altering the static and dynamic balance of the bow.

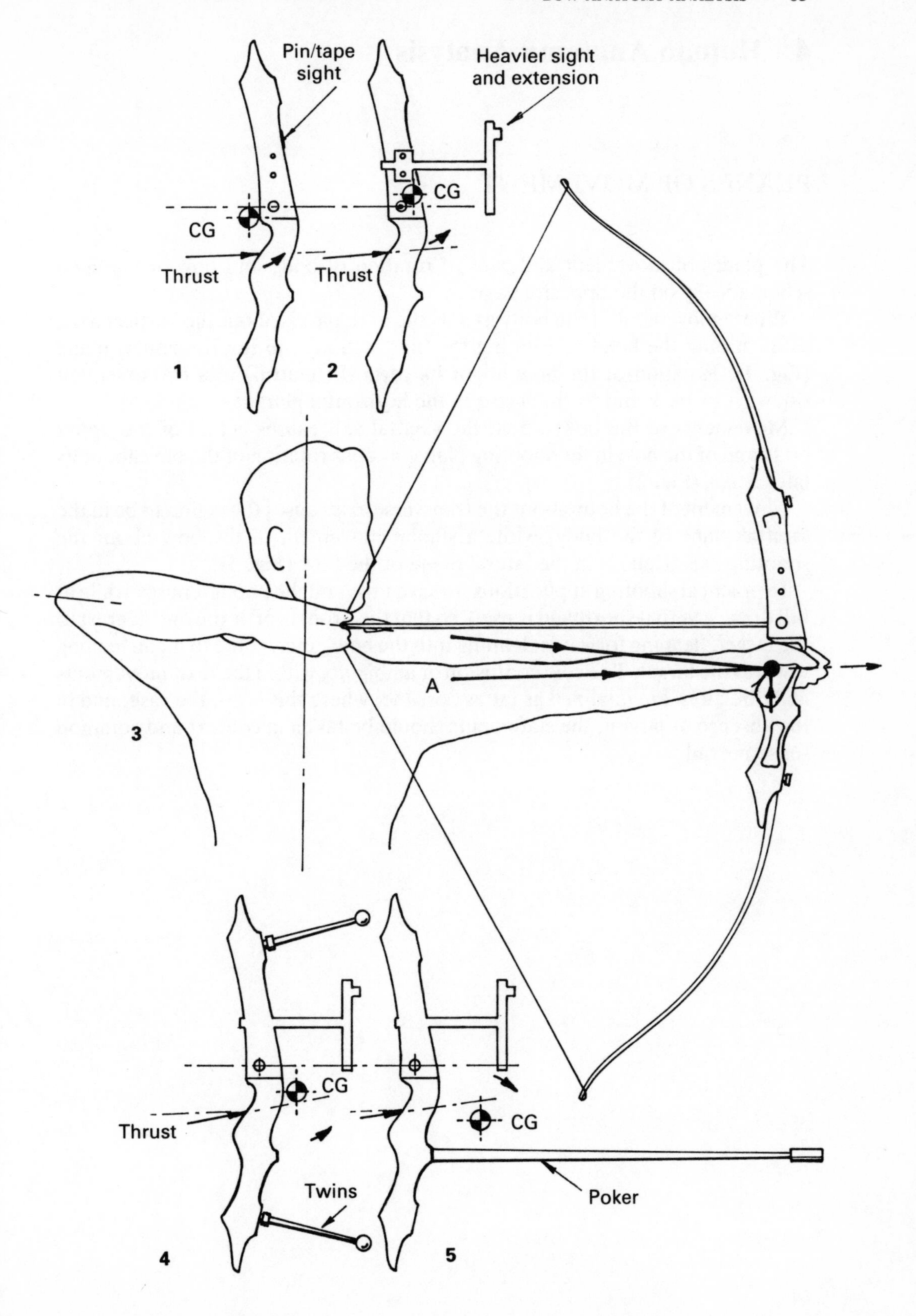
Pin/tape sight
Heavier sight and extension
CG
CG
Thrust
Thrust
1
2
A
3
CG
CG
Thrust
Twins
Poker
4
5

4 Human Anatomy Analysis

PLANES OF MOVEMENT

The planes of movement and axes of rotation of body and bow are defined schematically on the opposite page.

Where movement of the body as a whole or in part is about the vertical axis, as in turning the head or rotating the hips, action is in the horizontal plane (**Fig. 1**). Rotation of the bow about its vertical (neutral) axis or movement sideways or back and forth, is also in the horizontal plane.

Movements of the body about the sagittal axis causes action of the upper body and of the bow in the shooting plane, as does rotation of the bow about its lateral axis (**Fig. 2**).

Movement of the body about the transverse axis causes the action to be in the sagittal plane of the body, while a similar movement of the bow about the shooting axis (cant) is in the lateral plane of the bow (**Fig. 3**).

In practical shooting applications, to save time and the pupils' energy while at full draw, a verbal shorthand is used, so that the 'front foot' is the one nearest to the target, 'leaning forwards, leaning into the bow', etc., come to mean leaning towards the target. To avoid confusion or ambiguity within the text, movements and directions are qualified as far as possible; where this is not the case, and in the absence of jargon, the statements should be taken in context and common sense prevail.

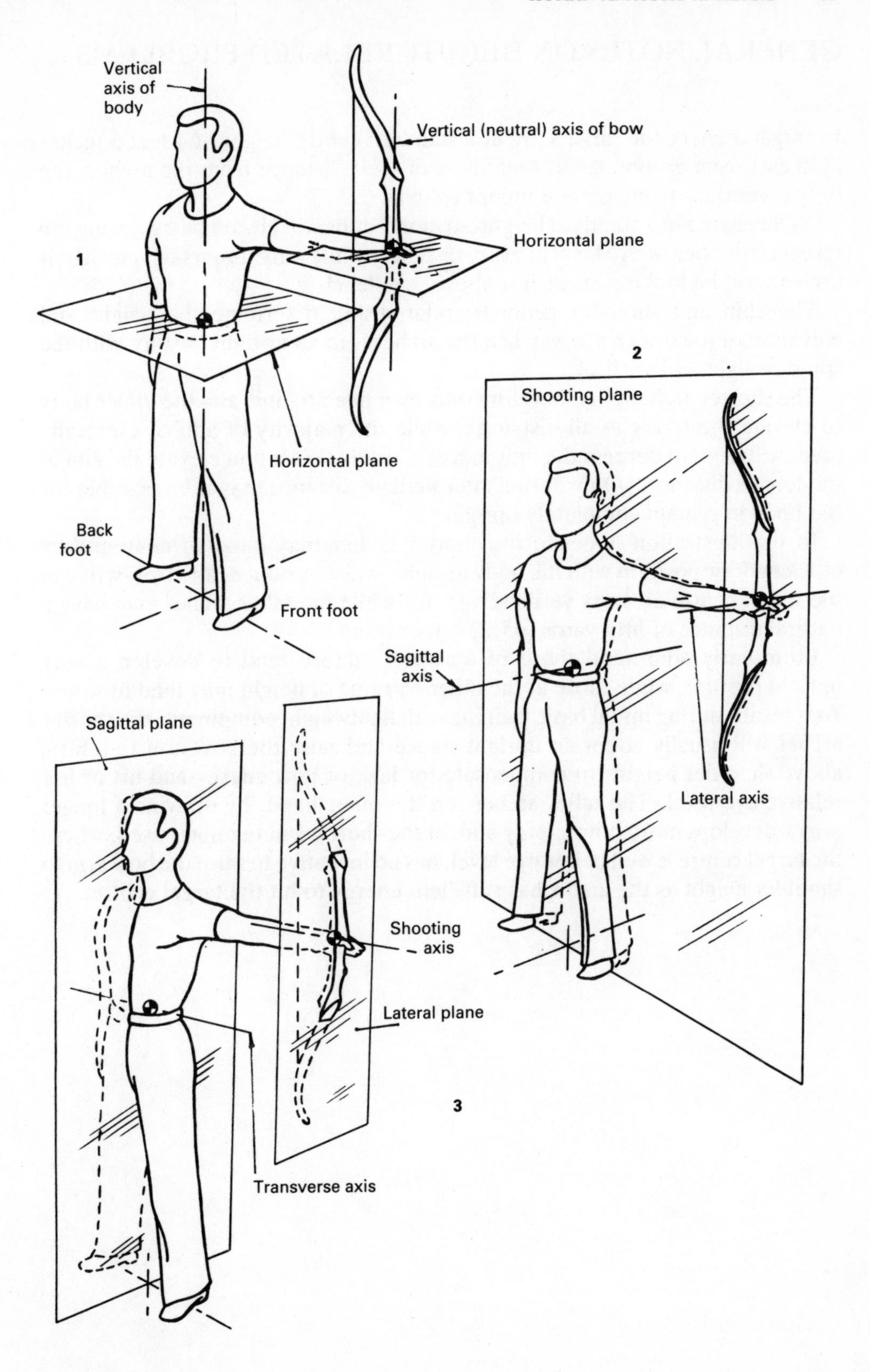
Vertical axis of body
Vertical (neutral) axis of bow
Horizontal plane
1
Horizontal plane
Back foot
Front foot
2
Shooting plane
Sagittal axis
Lateral axis
Sagittal plane
Shooting axis
Lateral plane
3
Transverse axis

GENERAL NOTES ON HEIGHT-RELATED PROBLEMS

In target archery the targets are at a standard centre height of 4 feet 3 inches (130 cm) from ground level, regardless of their distance from the archer, the only exceptions being certain indoor rounds.

Archers are not a standard height, so most adults will always be observing the target centre below eye level at every distance, while only juniors or wheelchair archers will be looking at, or just above, eye level.

The chin and shoulder geometry/relationship determine the height and elevation of the drawn arrow when the archer is in an upright posture with the spine straight and vertical.

The shorter archer may therefore only ever need to unit-aim the upper body to elevate the arrow at all distances, while the majority of adults, especially men, will need to depress the unit-aim at short distances and elevate the aim at the longer distances. Only at one intermediate distance may it be possible for the body to remain completely upright.

In the illustration opposite the shorter archer may have an anatomically efficient draw position with the body upright, which produces an arrow strike in the target centre at thirty yards (27.43 m), while the taller archer may have a natural distance of fifty yards (45.72 m), or more.

From early adulthood those of a shorter stature tend to develop a very upright posture, while those at the other extreme of height may tend to stoop. As a result, during initial basic training with lightweight equipment, the shorter archer will usually adopt an upright stance and raise the bow arm to a little above shoulder height, to compensate for lack of bow energy and his or her relative eye level. The taller archer, on the other hand, by drawing a longer arrow develops more bow energy and, at the short training ranges used, where the target centre is well below eye level, has no incentive to raise the bow arm to shoulder height as the arrow has sufficient energy to hit the target centre.

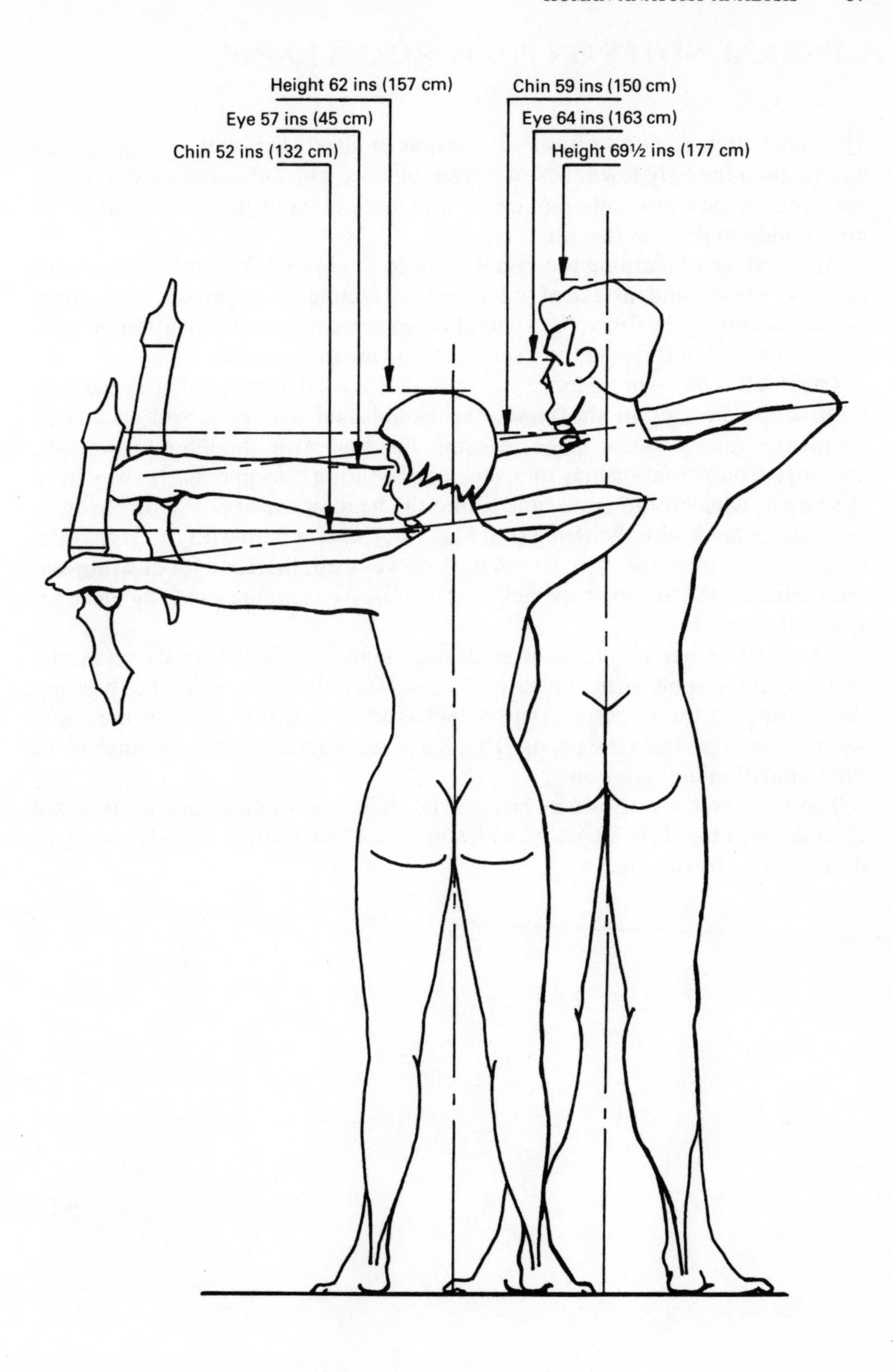
Height 62 ins (157 cm)
Eye 57 ins (45 cm)
Chin 52 ins (132 cm)
Chin 59 ins (150 cm)
Eye 64 ins (163 cm)
Height 69½ ins (177 cm)

GENERAL NOTES ON POSTURE COLLAPSE

The taller archer, during basic instruction at short distances, can generally handle the relatively low loads of a training bow with sufficient ease to make lowering the bow arm onto aim easier and more obvious than unit-aiming the upper body to depress the aim.

At this stage of learning the visual input to the brain takes precedence over the other senses, and instead of practising and feeling the alignment of the body as a whole during the draw, the archer becomes preoccupied with attempting to put each arrow in the gold, by every and any means possible.

The result is that when a more powerful bow is used, which can be as much as three times heavier in the hand, the established low bow arm technique frequently fails at some stage, causing the bow arm shoulder to collapse upwards. Compensation may then be made by tilting the upper body away from the target, while at the same time tilting the head in the opposite direction to establish contact with the string (see **Fig. 1**). Also common with this is that the load is on the arms, the draw length underdeveloped, there is a lot of string and body contact, the eye to arrow height is compressed and the resulting loose far from efficient.

Invariably, when this archer attempts unit-aiming at the longer distances, the 'S' bend in the spine at the lower end causes such discomfort that the hips are thrust towards the target, tilting the pelvis to reduce the angle of the spine where it emerges from the pelvis. This is a point to remember in the analysis of the foundation unit later on.

The same archer is shown in **Fig. 2** as he should be when aiming at the same distance as in **Fig. 1**, in a posture which he should have adopted and developed during basic instruction.

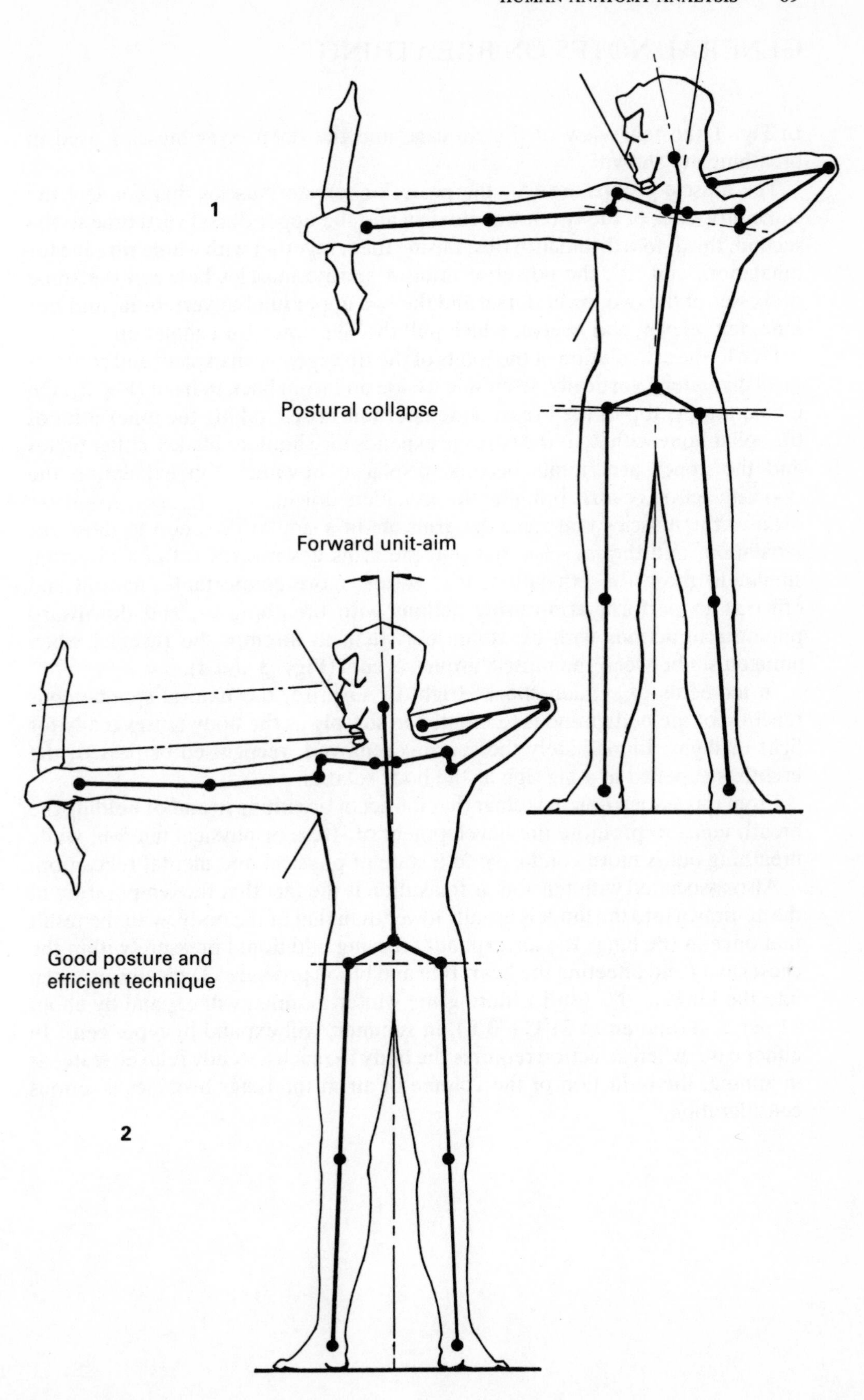
1
Postural collapse
Forward unit-aim
Good posture and
efficient technique
2

GENERAL NOTES ON BREATHING

In **Fig. 1** the rear view of the rib cage and the deep layer muscles used in breathing are shown.

The muscle groups are 'A', the posterior serrate muscles that connect the spine processes of the two lower cervical and the upper dorsal vertebrae to the second, third, fourth and fifth ribs, raising them together with whole rib cage for inhalation, and 'B', the posterior inferior serrate muscles between the spine processes of the two lower dorsal and the two upper lumbar vertebrae, and ribs nine, ten, eleven and twelve, which pull the ribs down for exhalation.

Due to the articulation of the joints of the rib cage, it can expand and contract in all diameters, vertically, from side to side and from back to front (**Fig. 2**). On inhalation the top of the breast bone (sternum) rises, taking the inner joint of the collar bone with it; as the rib cage expands the shoulder blades, collar bones and the upper arm joints become displaced upwards. On exhalation the opposite action occurs, bringing the shoulders down.

Since the muscles that raise the arms act in a similar direction to those for inhalation, and the muscles that pull the arms downwards act in a direction similar to those for exhalation, it is easier, more comfortable, natural and efficient to perform arm-raising actions with breathing in, and downward pulling arm actions with breathing out, than to attempt the reverse, when antagonism between the muscle groups occurs (**Figs. 3** and **4**).

In moments of sudden shock, fright or surprise, the natural spontaneous reaction of the body/mind is to breathe in sharply as the body tenses ready for fight or flight. Immediately the cause is removed, recognised or passed, the breath is expelled in a big sigh as the body relaxes.

From this association, it is clear that the act of breathing in and/or holding the breath tends to promote the development of stress or physical tension, while breathing out is more conducive to a state of physical and mental relaxation.

Also associated with tension or relaxation is the fact that the temperature of the air drawn into the lungs is usually lower than that of the body, with the result that once in the lungs the air expands, causing additional pressure within the chest cavity and affecting the heart rate and blood pressure. Typically air taken into the lungs at 0°C (30°F), during the winter months, will expand by about 12 per cent, and air at 21°C (70°F), in summer, will expand by 5 per cent. In either case, when an action requires the body to reach a steady relaxed state, as in aiming, the reduction of the volume of air in the lungs becomes a serious consideration.

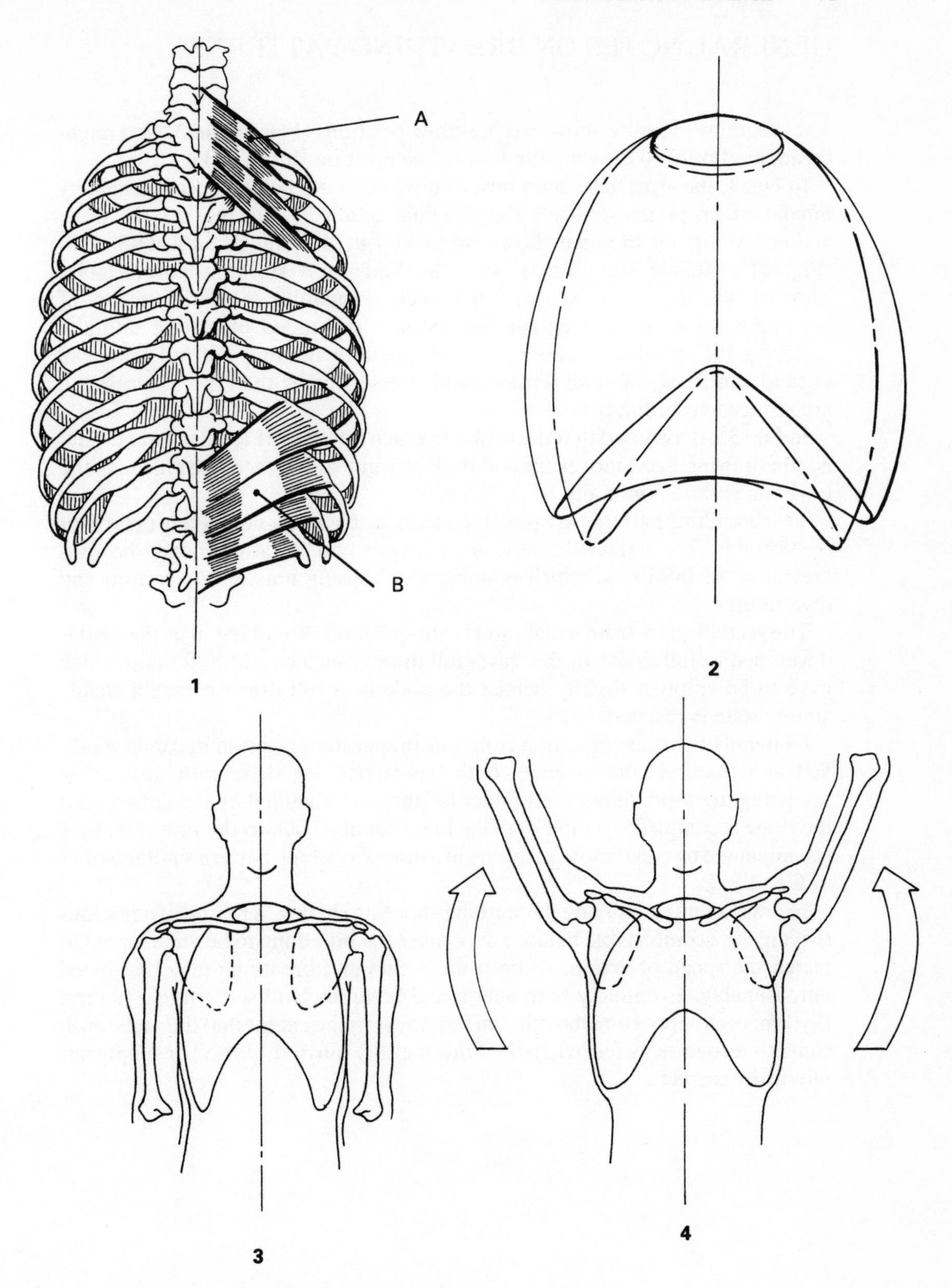
A
B
1
2
3
4

GENERAL NOTES ON BREATHING PATTERNS

The diagrams opposite show two pre-draw positions (**Figs. 1** and **3**) that might be adopted prior to drawing the bow to the position shown in **Fig. 2**.

In **Fig. 1**, the arms have been raised above shoulder height, accompanied by inhalation, in preparation for the dynamic action of drawing. As the draw action develops the breath is allowed to trickle out of the lungs, until at full draw (**Fig. 2**) a steady state exists with the lungs and rib cage comfortable. Throughout, the body actions have been compatible with the action of breathing, so no muscle antagonism occurs, the speed of action naturally matching the speed of breathing. Air retained in the lungs at full draw can expand harmlessly, and all tensions and stresses, other than those necessary, are reduced accordingly.

In **Fig. 3** it is assumed that the action to reach full draw (**Fig. 2**) is direct. That is, the drawing hand moves up and back straight to the face reference, as the bow arm is raised onto aim.

Two breathing patterns are possible, neither of which is competely natural or comfortable. The first is to breathe in, in this position, breathing out as the arms are raised to full draw, which is unnatural, causing muscle antagonism and discomfort.

The second starts from exhalation in this position, breathing in as the load is developed to full draw. In this case, full draw coincides with full lungs which have to be emptied slightly, whilst the body is at full draw, before a steady aiming state is reached.

Generally the drawing action from this preparation position becomes modified as a natural consequence: both hands rise together, with little draw occurring, to approximately shoulder height, accompanied by inhalation, and the draw is completed by the drawing hand coming back to the face reference accompanied by exhalation, resulting in a draw/breathing pattern similar to that of **Fig. 1**.

In developing an individual breathing/shooting rhythm, a period of conscious striving for a comfortable balance may cause the breathing to become forced to match the speed of action, or both the action and breathing may be slowed unreasonably. Eventually both action and breathing will settle into a natural rhythm, each supporting the other in harmony, to the extent that the archer will come to recognise by feel when the draw is either hurried, slowed or simply not physically correct.

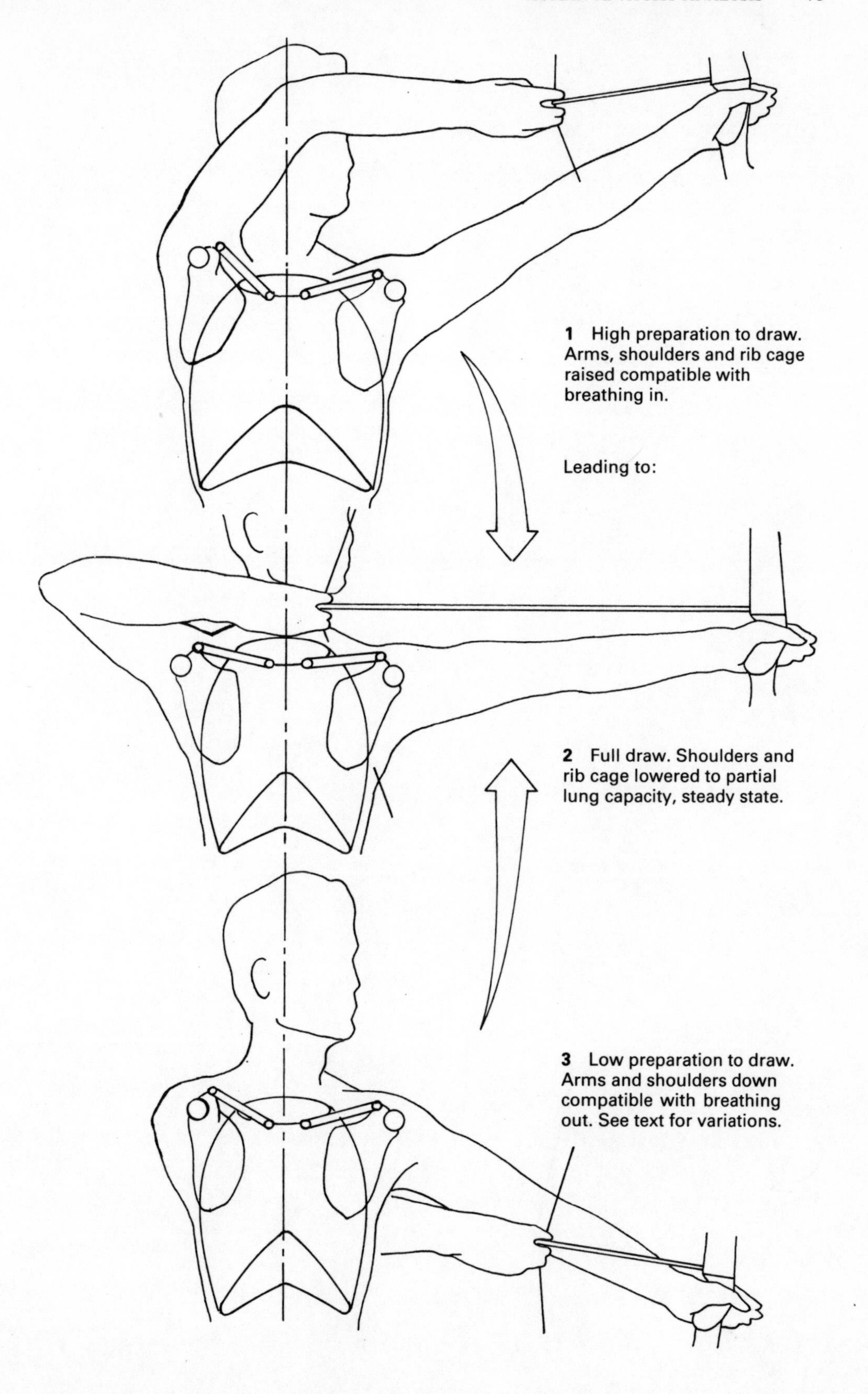

1 High preparation to draw. Arms, shoulders and rib cage raised compatible with breathing in.

Leading to:

2 Full draw. Shoulders and rib cage lowered to partial lung capacity, steady state.

3 Low preparation to draw. Arms and shoulders down compatible with breathing out. See text for variations.

PART TWO

TECHNIQUE ANALYSIS

Establishing the priorities

To decide which aspect of the physical skill of archery has priority over others is difficult, since all are important, interrelated and dependent one upon another. Ultimately the objective is to shoot 'good' arrows into a specific small area of a target at all distances, with the minimum of physical and mental effort.

Within the context of this book, 'good' arrows are those that leave the bow efficiently—that is, they are possessed of the maximum energy that can be transferred from the bow consistently so that each arrow behaves identically. For this situation to occur, the bow must also be possessed of and release the energy transferred to it from the archer's body efficiently and consistently, which in turn means that the archer must provide the energy required efficiently and consistently for every shot, with the minimum of wasted effort.

Since it is pointless to shoot any arrow that is less than 'good', no matter how well aimed physically or visually, it is the method or technique by which the biomechanical energy is developed, applied and released that takes first priority, under the heading of 'power unit analysis' with subdivisions 'power unit, bow hand analysis' and 'power unit, drawing hand analysis' and so on.

The second priority is the 'foundation unit' comprising the feet, legs and hips, which provide the support, direction and elevation of the power unit, and lastly the 'confirmation unit' comprising the head, neck, jaw and eyes, which, in physical relationship to the drawn bow and power/foundation units, visually confirms the precise aim and mentally instructs and monitors the physical performance.

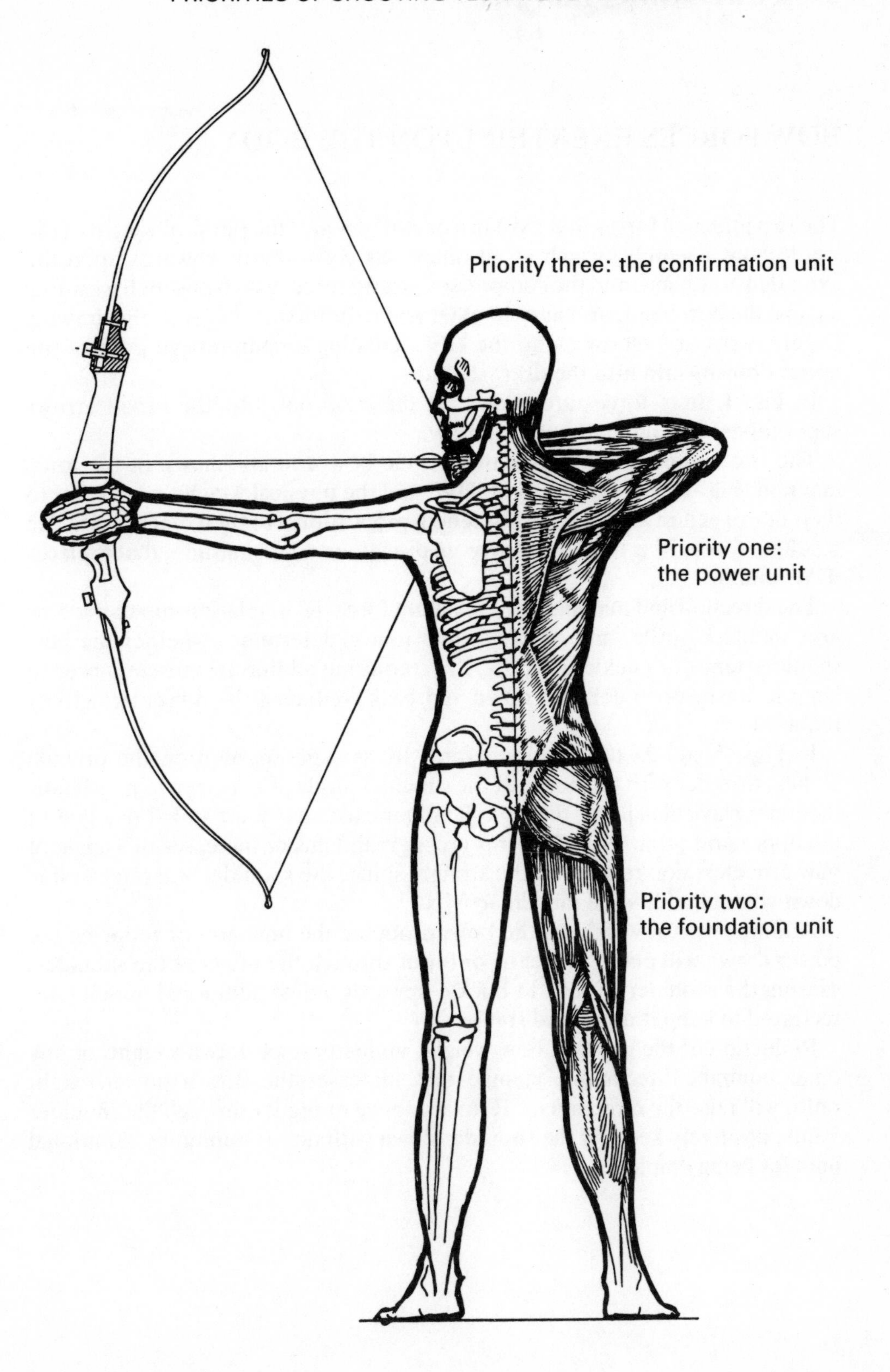
PRIORITIES OF SHOOTING TECHNIQUE ANALYSIS
Priority three: the confirmation unit
Priority one:
the power unit
Priority two:
the foundation unit

5 Power Unit Analysis

BOW FORCES EXERTED UPON THE BODY

The two principal forces that exist in a drawn bow are: the physical weight of the whole bow assembly, which at all times acts vertically downwards upon the extended bow hand, and the compressive drawn force, which pushes backwards against the bow hand, arm and shoulder and pulls forwards against the drawing fingers, wrist and elbow along the DFL, creating a compressive push of the upper drawing arm into the draw shoulder.

In **Fig. 1** these forces are shown, in direction only, by the broad arrows superimposed on an archer at full draw.

The two component forces acting on the bow arm are shown in the force diagram (**Fig. 2**): the draw weight 'DW' and the physical weight 'w' parallel to their line of action in **Fig. 1** and to a length proportional to their magnitude. The resultant force 'R' is the single force, in direction and magnitude, that replaces 'DW' and 'w'.

The direction and magnitude of resultant force 'R' in relationship to the bow arm shoulder girdle, and its bones and joints, determines whether the bow shoulder tends to buckle upwards, thus requiring additional muscle power to keep it down, or to collapse down and back, reducing the muscular activity required.

In **Figs. 3** and **3a** this resultant force 'R' is superimposed on the original archer, together with the bones of the shoulder girdle, and is seen to pass below the inner clavicular joint, through the outer clavicular joint and above that of the upper arm joint. Providing this archer maintains or increases this angle of bow arm elevation relative to the straight spine, the shoulder will tend to stay down without additional muscle activity.

Adding physical weight to the bow, dropping the bow arm or reducing the power drawn will place 'R' below or lower through the joints of the shoulder, causing the shoulder to tend to buckle upwards unless additional muscles are recruited to keep it down and stable.

Reduction of the physical bow weight, an increase of drawn weight, or any other equipment/technique change that increases the drawn power/weight ratio, will raise the direction of 'R' to act above or higher through the shoulder joints, positively keeping the shoulder down with no, or minimum, additional muscles being employed.

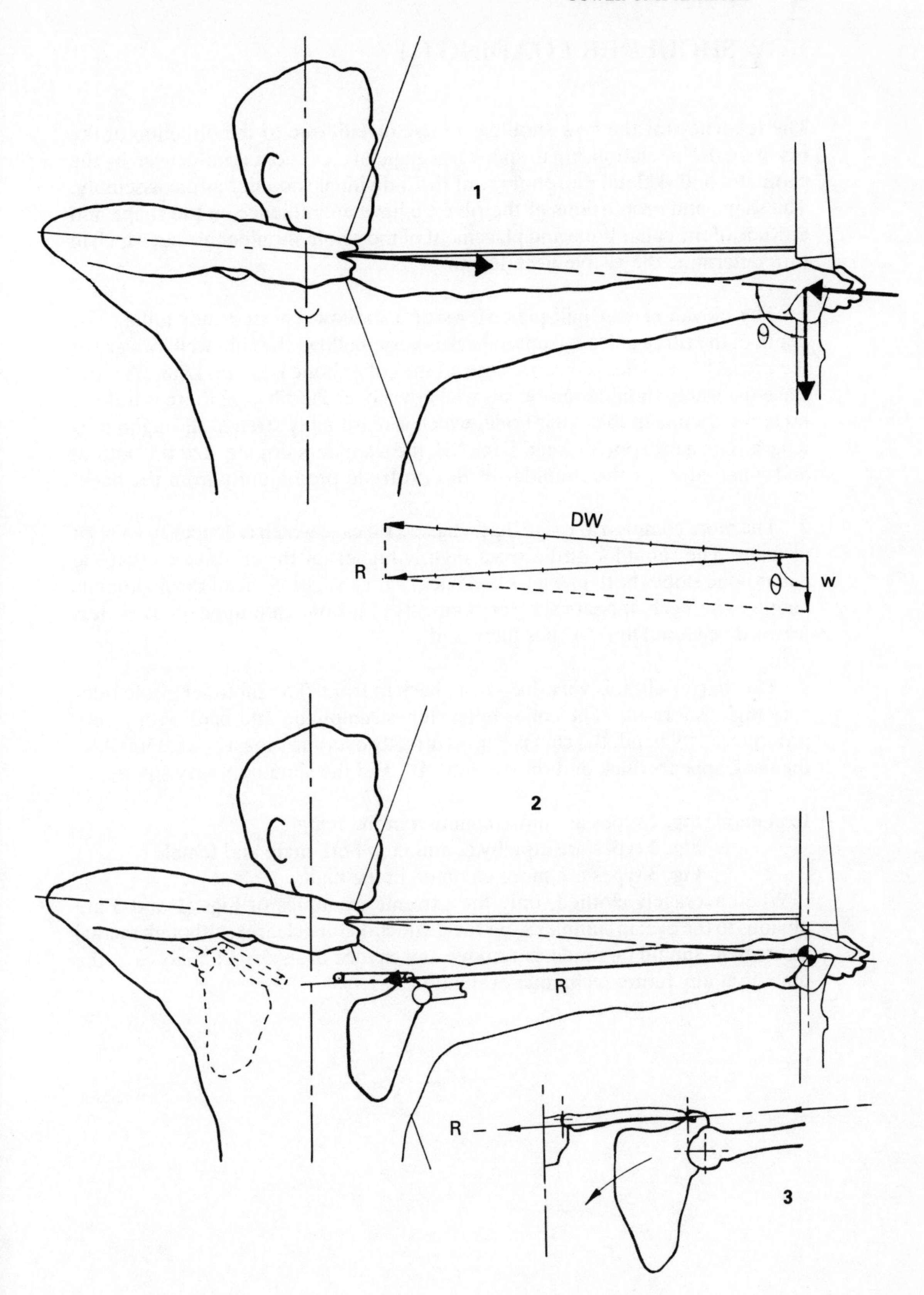
1
DW
R
θ
W
2
R
R
3

BOW SHOULDER LOADING (1)

The tendency for the bow shoulder to rise or fall, due to the direction of the resultant 'R' in relationship to spine/arm angle of elevation, is influenced by the geometry and skeletal morphology of the individual shoulder girdle assembly. The shape and proportions of the rib cage have an influence on the shape and attitude of the collar bone and placement of the whole shoulder girdle, which in turn determine the visible neck length.

1 The elevation and half-plan views of a 'hollow'-chested individual. The depth of the rib cage from front to back is very shallow, the chin well forward of the breast bone. The backward slope of the collar bone is small, Dim. 'A', and since the whole shoulder girdle sits well down over the rib cage there is little or no upward slope to the collar bone, which is reasonably straight throughout its length. The neck appears long, Dim. 'B', the shoulders sloping, and the bottom and inner edges of the shoulder blades protrude prominently from the back.

2 The more common average 'flat'-chested rib cage which is deeper from back to front. The shoulder girdle rides slightly higher on the rib cage so that the collar bone slopes both upwards and back, with a slight 'S' bend throughout its length. The neck appears shorter, Dim. 'B', and the chin appears to be less forward because Dim. 'A' has increased.

3 The 'barrel' chest is very deep from back to front. The shoulder girdle rides very high as a result. The collar bone slopes steeply up and back with a very pronounced 'S' bend, the chin is almost directly over the breast bone, Dim. 'A', the neck appears thick and short, Dim. 'B', and the shoulders very square.

In general, **Fig. 1** types are more common in the female.
Fig. 2 types are equally common in both male and female.
Fig. 3 types are more common in the male.

When averagely clothed, only the extreme examples of **Figs. 1** and **3** are obvious to the eye; in summer wear the distinctions are clearer, although tactual assessment should be made to remove any chance of incorrect analysis at the time or at any future technique evaluation.

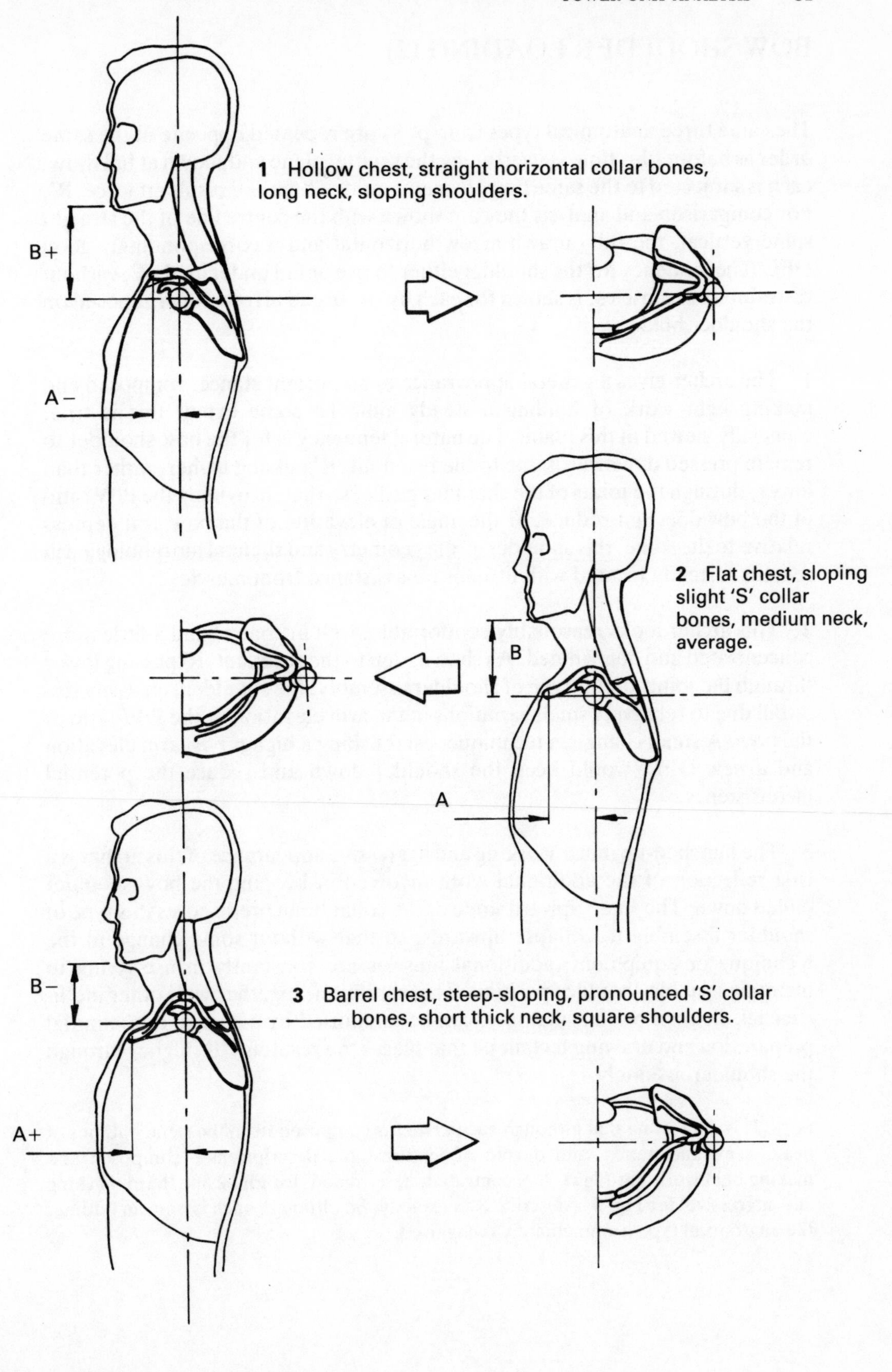
B+
A−
1 Hollow chest, straight horizontal collar bones, long neck, sloping shoulders.
2 Flat chest, sloping slight 'S' collar bones, medium neck, average.
B
A
B−
A+
3 Barrel chest, steep-sloping, pronounced 'S' collar bones, short thick neck, square shoulders.

BOW SHOULDER LOADING (2)

The same three anatomical types from p. 81 are repeated opposite in the same order as before, this time viewed along the sagittal plane and shown at full draw; each is subjected to the same power/weight ratio of bow and resultant force 'R'. For comparison and analysis they are shown with the centre line of the straight spine vertical, the fully drawn arrow horizontal and a correspondingly good DFL. The tendency for the shoulder either to rise or fall under load 'R', without restraint from muscles, is shown for each by the broad arrows superimposed on the shoulder blade.

1 The archer gives a general appearance of an upright stance, composed and making light work of holding a steady aim. To some extent this is true, especially viewed in this plane. The natural tendency is for the bow shoulder to remain pressed downwards due to the resultant 'R' passing higher, rather than lower, through the joints of the shoulder girdle, so that, providing the P/W ratio of the bow does not reduce, or the angle of elevation of the bow arm depress relative to the spine, this shoulder girdle geometry and skeletal morphology will remain correctly located with little or no assistance from muscles.

2 This archer looks reasonably comfortable, well in control and a little more concentrated and determined. As shown, due to the resultant 'R' passing lower through the joints of this type of shoulder assembly, the shoulder can easily rise or fall due to relatively small variations in the arm elevation or the P/W ratio of the bow. A small change in technique, establishing a higher bow arm elevation and a new DFL, would keep the shoulder down and reduce the potential inconsistency.

3 The hunched-up, hard-working and aggressive appearance of this archer is a true reflection of the additional work involved in keeping the bow shoulder pulled down. The steep upward slope of the collar bone predisposes this type of shoulder assembly to collapse upwards, so that without some change in the technique or equipment, additional muscles are constantly in use trying to maintain a stable shoulder position. This condition, together with other inefficiencies dictated by this anatomy, can be minimised by a change in the initial preparation and drawing technique that places the resultant 'R' higher through the shoulder assembly.

NOTE: It is interesting that although each archer is composed from the same outlines of head, arms and hands, and devoid of features, the descriptions—'composed and making light work' for **Fig. 1**, 'concentrated, determined' for **Fig. 2** and 'hard-working and aggressive' for **Fig. 3**—describe each exactly. So although each is only an outline, the anatomical type is immediately recognised.

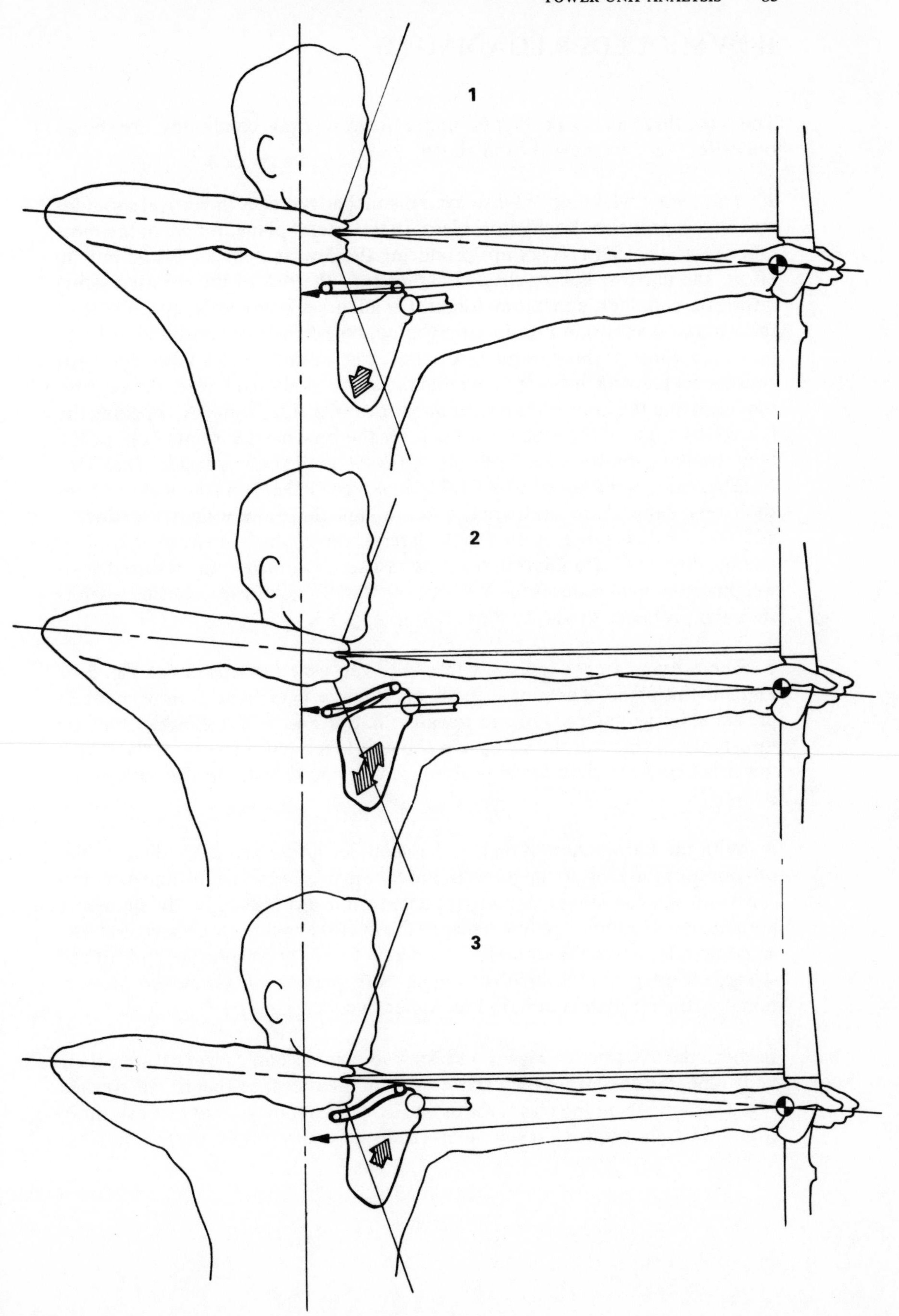
1
2
3

BOW SHOULDER LOADING (3)

The same three anatomical types, under the same draw conditions, are shown opposite, this time viewed from above.

1 This archer who on p. 83 displayed distinct advantages in vertical shoulder stability, is prone to shoulder problems in the lateral plane, for when the most efficient vertical DFL is set up, producing the lowest joint loads and muscle effort, the narrow, hollow-chested archer runs the risk of the released string hitting the shoulder, upper arm, forearm or all three. Frequently, one or both of the variations shown in **Fig. 1a** are adopted, consciously or subconsciously, to avoid repetition of this painful experience. The turned head is taken forwards over the feet, giving the impression that the archer is about to overbalance, with the result that the draw is shortened on the drawing side, Dim. 'A', opening the horizontal angle of the elbow joint (θ). Or the bow hand is rotated out of the bow, cranking the wrist and reducing the draw on the bow arm side, Dim. 'B'. In either case, as the line of effort, DFL, is moved farther from the joints of both shoulders, bow elbow and wrist, even though the draw weight is reduced, additional muscle power is used in the lateral plane, which, apart from wasting energy, disposes these joints to react inconsistently. Further, the reduced draw weight component reduces the P/W ratio so that 'R' acts lower, causing vertical shoulder problems similar to those in Fig. 2, p. 83.

2 The average archer can show tendencies to vary towards either **Fig. 1** or **Fig. 3** in this plane of action, as in the previous vertical plane of movement. If the shoulder geometry is biased towards that of **Fig. 1**, the shoulder may be thrust into the path of the string and show little tendency to rise; if the bias is towards **Fig. 3** the shoulder may rise but never be thrust into the path of the string.

3 With the barrel-chested archer the shoulder girdle geometry dictates the proximity of the DFL to the joints of the shoulders, and while the line of action can be set up to be consistent and as efficient as the morphology of the shoulders permits, it will seldom approach that of the average or hollow-chested archers; consequently, while the shoulder is unlikely to be thrust into the path of the string, the total muscle involvement in both planes will always be proportionately higher than in either of the other two.

Because the extremes of **Figs. 1** and **3** are so obvious and consistent with their body type, the analysis of their shooting form is easier than that of the average **Fig. 2** archer, where the bias towards one or the other may occur inconsistently from shot to shot and as a result, unless analysed anatomically, defy correction.

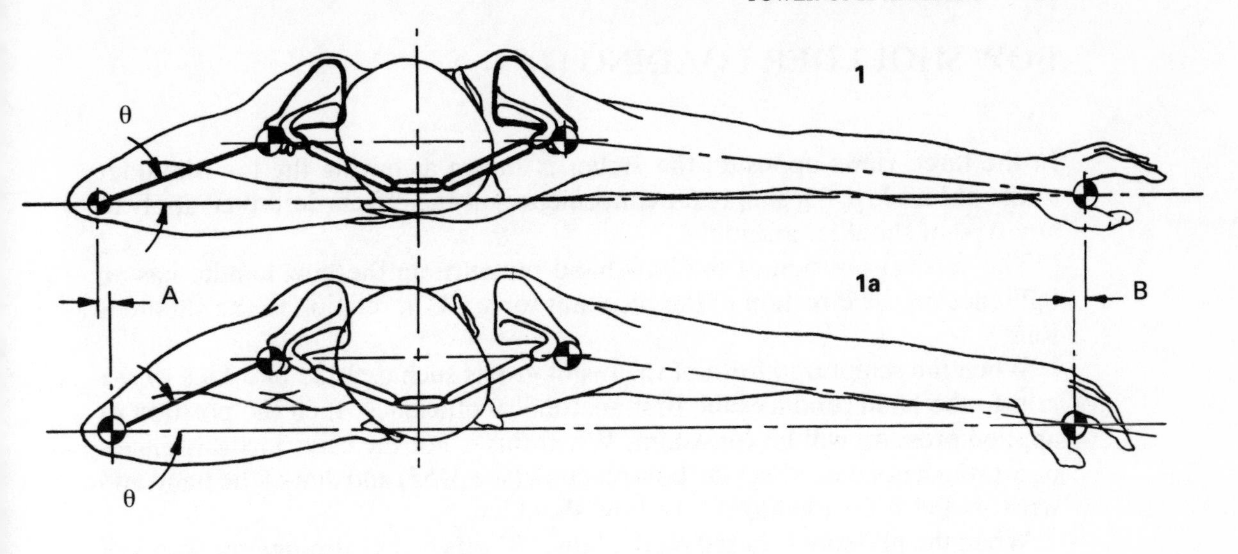
1
θ
1a
A
B
θ

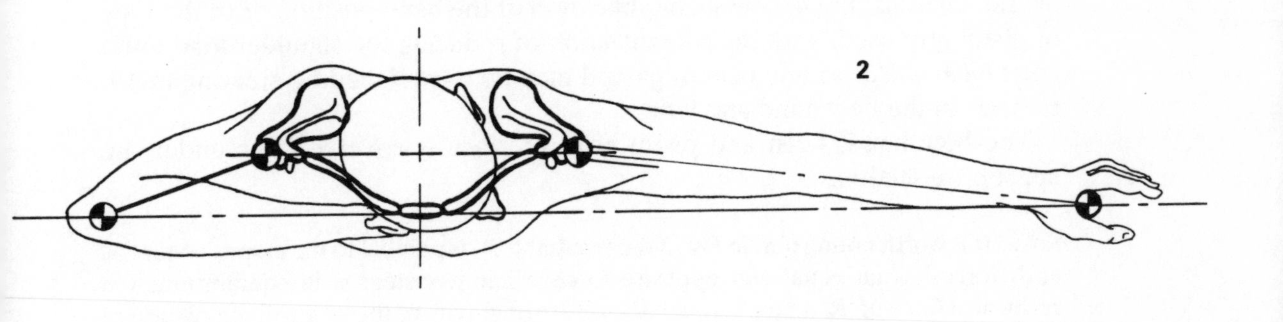
2

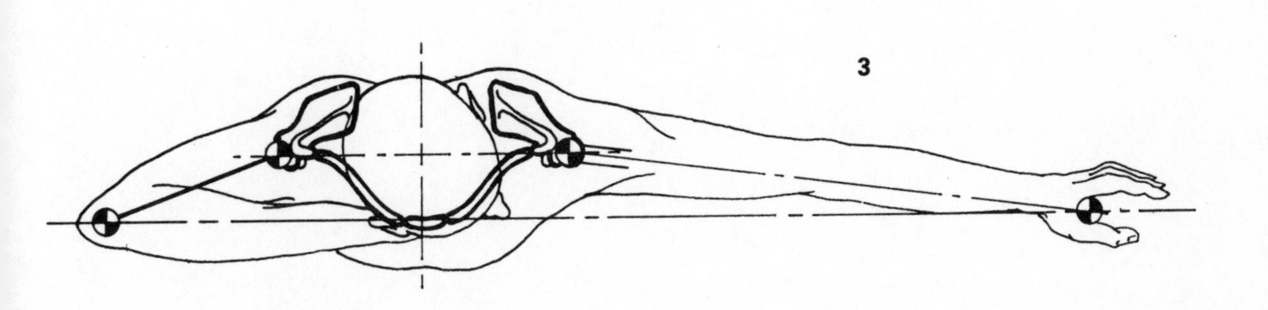
3

BOW SHOULDER LOADING (4)

In the three views opposite, the archer is shown as having the low shoulder girdle of Fig. 1, p. 83, simply for convenience, as the effects described apply to any type of shoulder assembly.

The vertical position of the bow hand pressure on the bow handle has an influence on the direction of the resultant force 'R' in relation to the shoulder joint.

When the sculptured form of the pistol grip is such that the interface of the grip to the hand produces the best anatomical efficiency, then the position of applied pressure will be consistent. When this is not the case, inconsistencies occur which not only affect the bow reaction (see p. 57) and that of the hand and wrist, but also the loading on the bow shoulder.

When the pressure is raised on the bow, 'R' acts higher through the joints of the shoulder, tending to assist in keeping it down and stable; as the pressure is lowered, so 'R' also acts lower, tending to raise the shoulder (**Figs. 1**, **2** and **3**).

While this effect upon the bow shoulder load must be considered as part of an overall analysis, the *deliberate* modification of the hand position or of the type of pistol grip used, with the *sole intention* of reducing the shoulder load only, *must be avoided*, as any benefit gained may be outweighed by creating inefficiencies in the bow hand and wrist.

The bow hand, wrist and pistol grip interface is covered later under the approprite section.

NOTE: It is worth noting that in **Fig. 3** the resultant 'R' is parallel to the arrow, so that as each force has an equal and opposite force, when a system is in equilibrium, the reciprocal force of 'R' acting through the centre of gravity of the bow will, on release of the string, move the bow straight forwards parallel to the intended path of the arrow (see arrow 'A', Fig. 3, p. 63). The reciprocal of 'R' in **Figs. 1** and **2** opposite, however, would act in an upward direction and deflect the arrow accordingly.

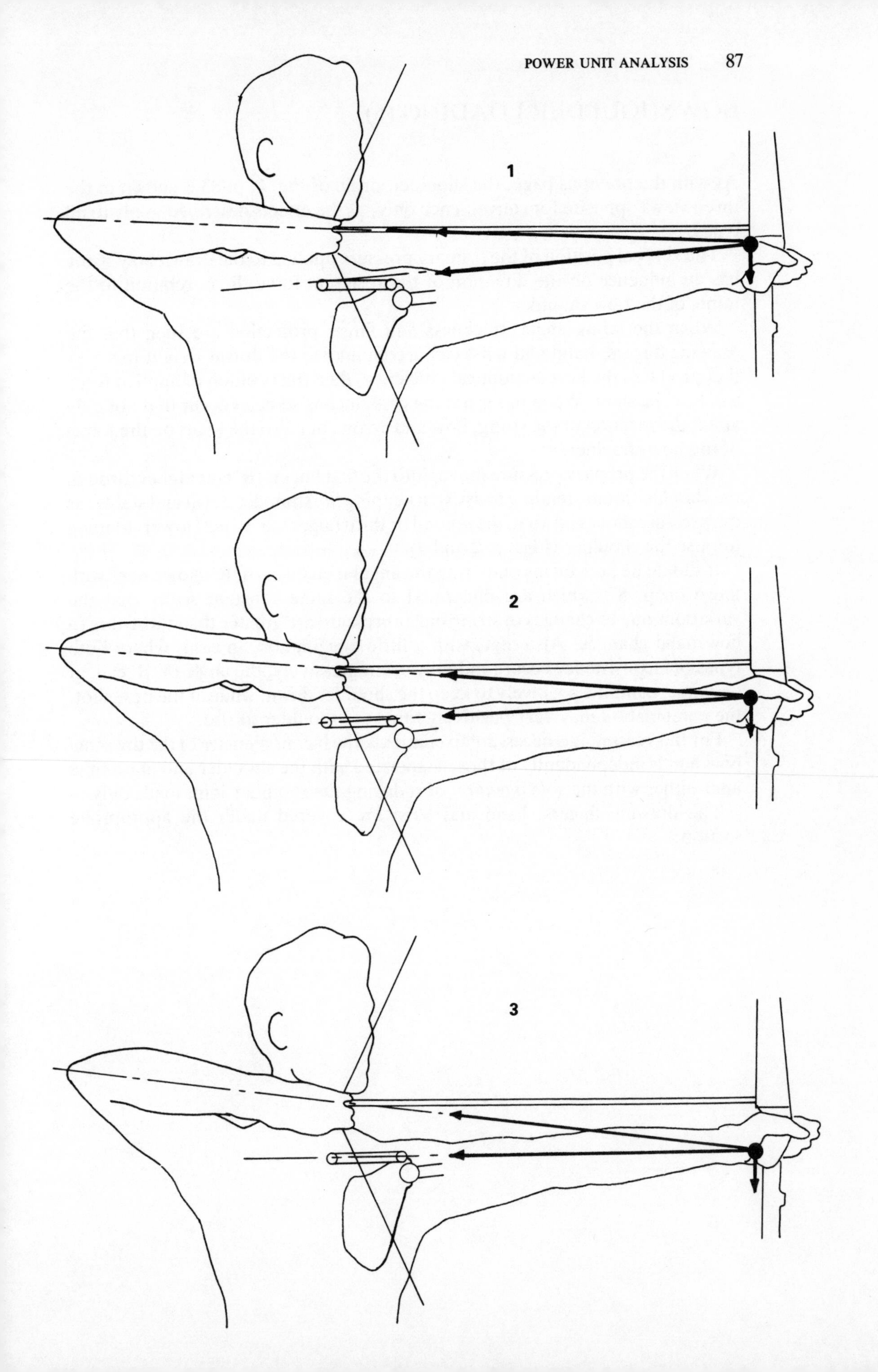
1
2
3

BOW SHOULDER LOADING (5)

As with the previous page, the shoulder girdle of Fig. 1, p. 83 is shown in the three views opposite for convenience only, as the effects described apply to all types.

The vertical position of the primary pressure applied to the drawn bow string has an influence on the direction of the resultant force 'R' in relation to the joints of the bow shoulder.

When the string angle, thickness and finger protection are such that the drawing fingers, hand and wrist can accommodate the drawn weight in a way that produces the best anatomical efficiency, then the position of applied force will be consistent. When this is not the case, inconsistencies occur that not only affect the reaction of the string, bow and arrow, but also the loads on the joints of the bow shoulder.

When the primary pressure moves into the first finger, 'R' acts higher through the shoulder joints, tending to assist in keeping the shoulder down and stable; as the pressure moves down to the second or third finger, so 'R' acts lower, tending to raise the shoulder (**Figs. 1**, **2** and **3**).

It should be noticed in comparing the angular changes of 'R' shown here with those on p. 87, which are illustrated to the same constant scale, that the variations due to changes of string finger pressure are greater than those due to bow hand changes. Also that, with a little imagination, in cases where both types of inconsistency occur randomly or progressively, the angle of 'R' can, at one time, combine positively to keep the shoulder down, while at the next shot, the combination may very positively force the shoulder to rise.

For this reason, it is necessary to eliminate the inconsistencies of the drawing/bow hands independently of those associated with the shoulder and at no time alter either with the *sole intention* of reducing the shoulder joint loads only.

The drawing fingers, hand and wrist are covered under the appropriate section.

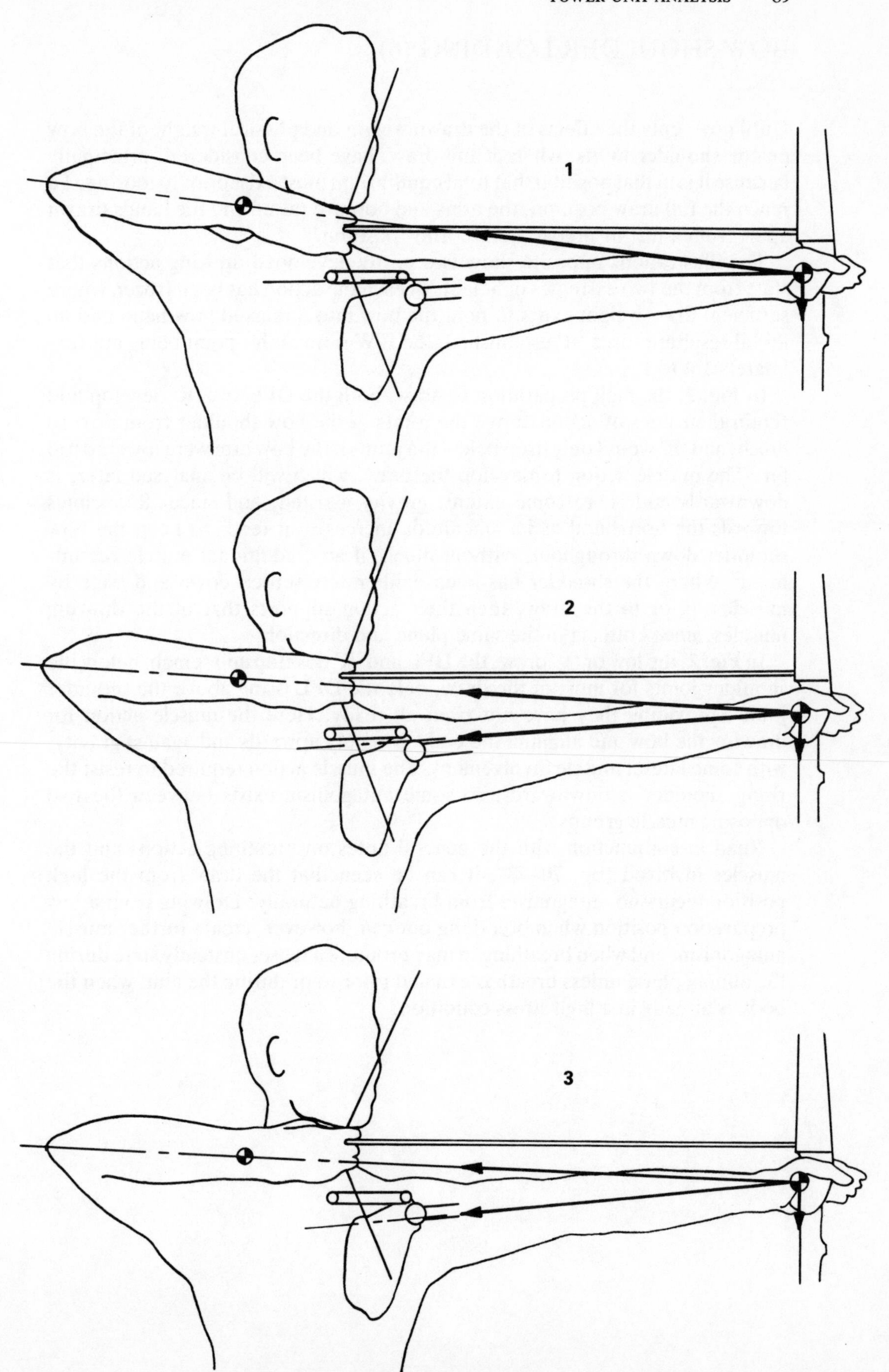
1
2
3

BOW SHOULDER LOADING (6)

Until now, only the effects of the drawn weight and physical weight of the bow on the shoulder joints, when at full draw, have been considered, principally because it is in that position that total equilibrium must exist prior to loosing. To reach the full draw position, the arms and bow are raised and the hands drawn apart from a rest or preparation to draw position.

The illustrations opposite show two partly developed drawing actions that start from the two extremes of height. In each the action has been frozen where sufficient draw weight exists to hold the bow into a relaxed bow hand and an initial resultant force 'R' established, the P/W ratio at this point being approximately 1.4 to 1.

In **Fig. 1**, the high preparation to draw, both the DFL and 'R' develop and retain their lines of action above the joints of the bow shoulder from start to finish, and 'R' would only drop below the joints if the bow arm were lowered too far. The muscle action to develop the draw, which will be analysed later, is downwards and is, to some extent, gravity assisted, and since 'R' inclines towards the horizontal as its magnitude increases, it tends to keep the bow shoulder down throughout, without much, if any, additional muscle recruitment. Where the shoulder has been deliberately settled down and back by muscles, prior to the draw, then their action supports that of the drawing muscles, since both act in the same plane and direction.

In **Fig. 2**, the low or 'V' draw, the DFL and 'R' develop and remain below the shoulder joints for most of the draw, only the DFL rising above the shoulder joints, providing they have not risen all ready. Here the muscle action for drawing the bow and aligning the body is mainly upwards and against gravity, with some lateral muscle involvement. The muscle action required to resist the rising shoulder is downwards, so some antagonism exists between the two opposing muscle groups.

Read in conjunction with the general notes on breathing actions and the muscles involved (pp. 70–73), it can be seen that the draw from the high position incurs no antagonism from breathing naturally. Drawing from a low preparation position when breathing out can, however, create further muscle antagonism, and when breathing in may promote a tense, unsteady state during the aiming phase unless breath is exhaled prior to or during the aim, when the body is already in a high stress condition.

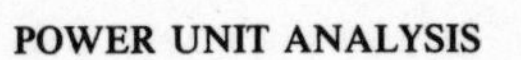

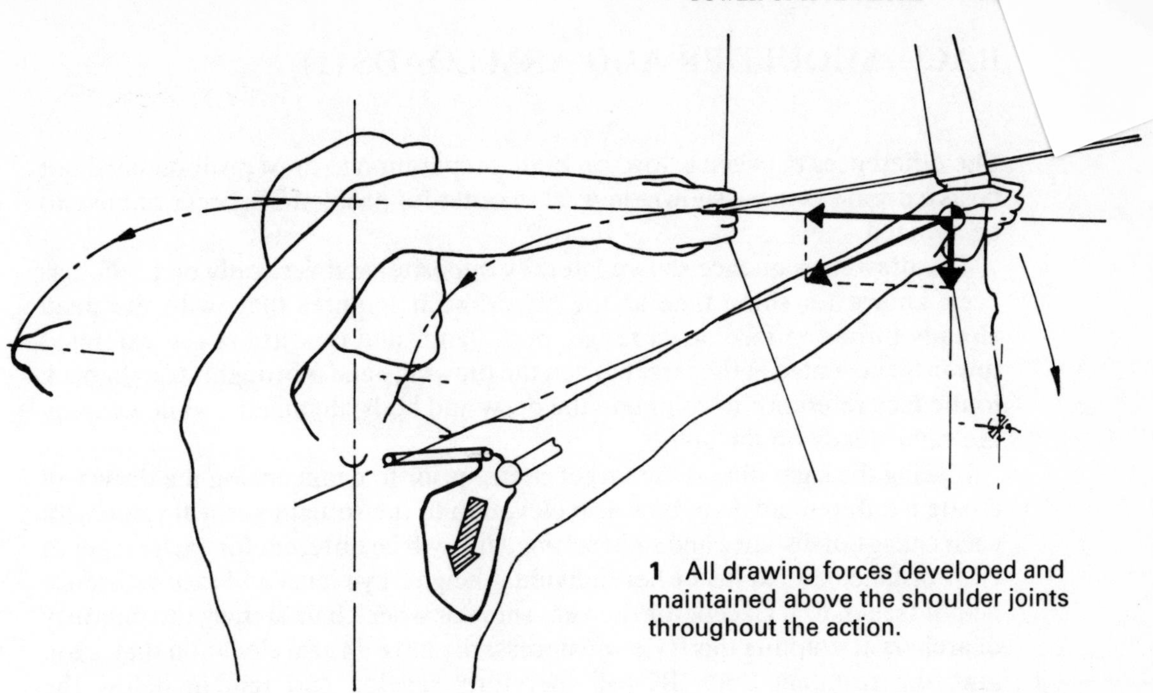

1 All drawing forces developed and maintained above the shoulder joints throughout the action.

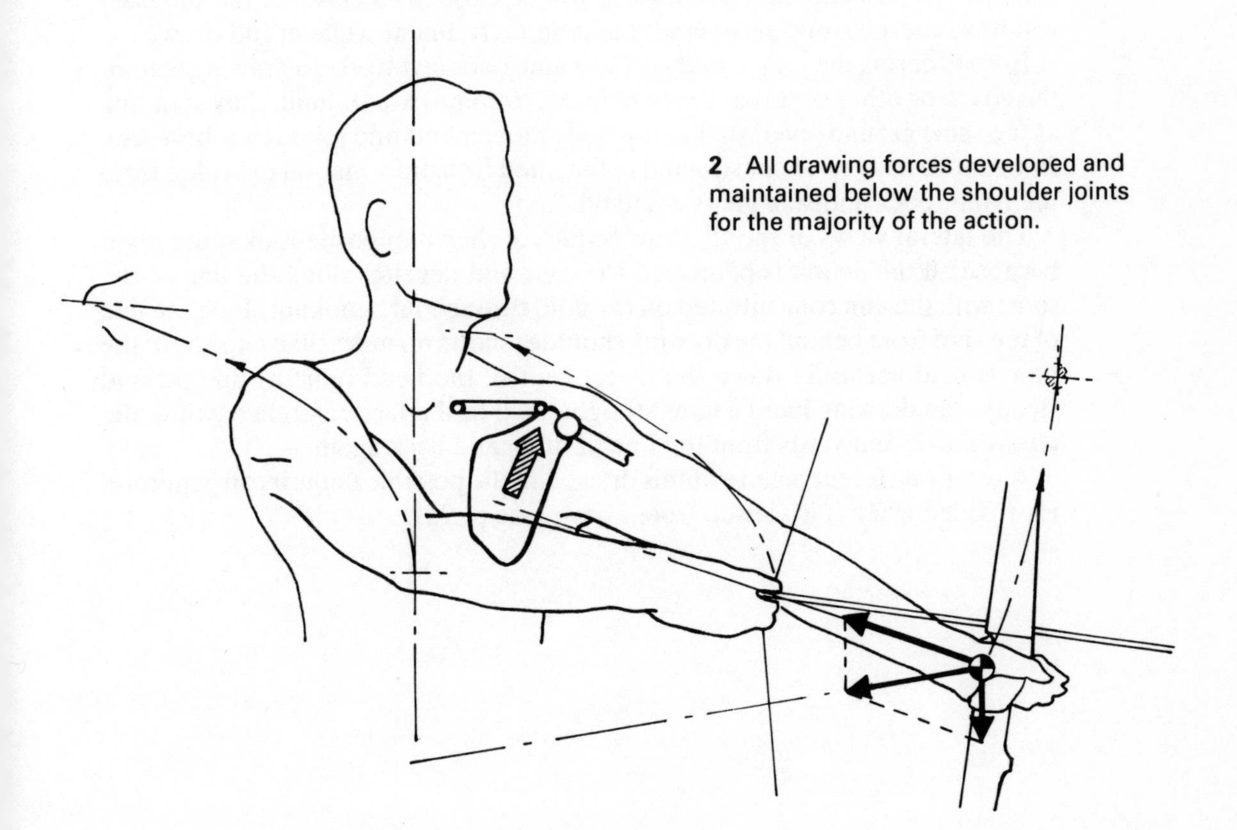

2 All drawing forces developed and maintained below the shoulder joints for the majority of the action.

BACK, SHOULDER AND ARM LOADS (1)

The differences between a 'low' or 'high' preparation to draw position need not be as extreme as those shown on p. 91 in order for problems to occur or have to be avoided.

The drawing sequence shown laterally opposite, and vertically on p. 95, has been known for some time as the 'T' draw. It requires that, with the head already turned to face down range, both hands and bow are raised extended towards and aimed at the target. Then the drawing hand is brought straight back to the face reference to complete the draw and body alignment, while keeping the sight steady on the gold.

Placing the sight pin on the target centre prior to commencing the draw will create a different angle of bow arm elevation to the straight vertical spine with each change of distance and sight setting, and will be different for each archer at each distance due to his or her individual height, eye level and face reference height (see p. 67). Except for the very short or wheelchair archer, the majority of archers attempting this style will necessarily have an arm elevation that is too low; the resultant load 'R' will therefore develop and remain below the shoulder joint throughout, by which time either the muscles recruited to stabilise the bow shoulder downwards will be close to collapse, or the shoulder will have risen beyond recovery by muscle recruitment while at full draw.

In considering the joints, body actions and loads involved in a drawing action, the coach or other observer's viewpoint is, to some extent, limited by standing at the same ground level, so that the body movements and joint loads best seen from above have to be constructed in the mind from information provided from the front, back and side views available.

The lateral views of the 'T' draw sequence shown opposite look quite good because all the action is perceived to occur and develop along the line of the shot, with the aim concentrated on the gold throughout. Looking along the line of the shot from behind the drawing shoulder shows no more than expected: the bow is held vertically down the target centre, the head remains upright and steady, the drawing hand comes straight back to the face reference, while the elbow moves outwards from the line of draw and back again.

A totally different picture of this draw, and the possible faults it can generate, is provided when it is viewed from above (see p. 95).

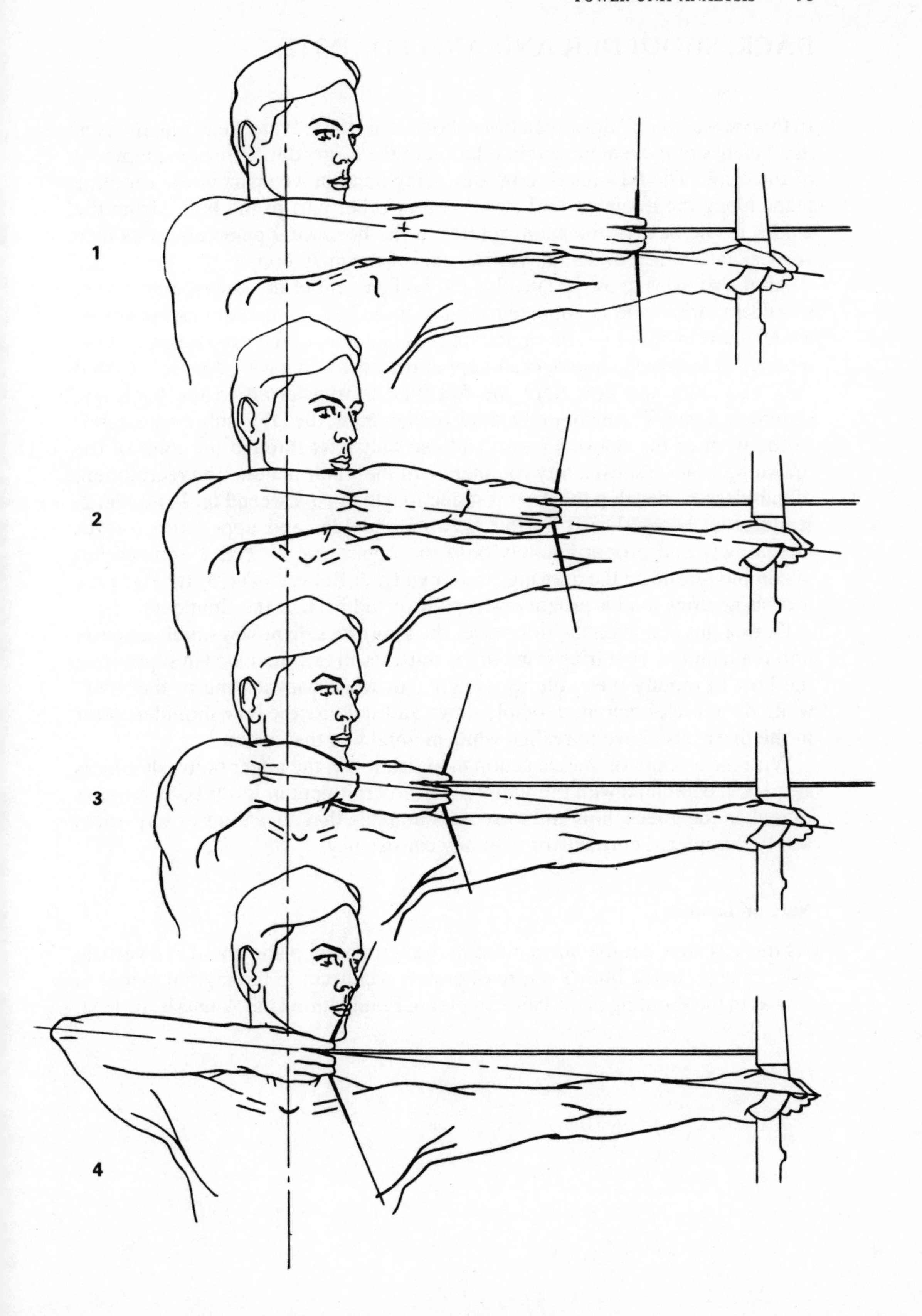
1
2
3
4

BACK, SHOULDER AND ARM LOADS (2)

In this view of the 'T' draw seen from above, only the feet and head remain fixed in all planes of movement and in relation to the target during the development of the draw. The bow hand, bow and string hand move apart in the shooting plane along the intended DFL, while every other part of the body, from the ankles to the base of the skull, rotates in the horizontal plane about its own vertical axis, which orbits the vertical axis of the main body.

All the muscles in use are involved in realignment of the knees, hips, torso, shoulders, arms, and in counter-rotation of the head to maintain its position, while others in both forearms maintain the alignment of the hands. Some of the muscles of the back, shoulders and upper drawing arm have a dual role in that they also draw the bow until the full load is transferred to the back and shoulders alone. Throughout the draw realignment, the DFL only ever extends to the wrist of the drawing hand, and can only pass through the joint of the drawing elbow on satisfactory completion of the whole action. The recruitment of muscles that develop the draw is sequential in that between **Fig. 1** and **Fig. 2**. It starts by being shared by the drawing shoulder and upper arm, moves increasingly and proportionately onto the upper arm by **Fig. 2** and reaches maximum torque on the drawing elbow by **Fig. 3**. Between **Fig. 3** and **Fig. 4** the increasing draw load is progressively transferred back to the shoulders.

During this action on the draw side, the bow arm side moves simultaneously into realignment, requiring some of the muscles already involved in supporting the bow to modify their role to realignment while contributing to the draw, while the muscles recruited to hold down and stabilise the bow shoulder, prior to the draw, also have to realign while maintaining that action.

With the amount of muscle action modification in the upper body, shoulders and arms, combined with the simultaneous recruitment of lower body muscles to realign the knees, hips and torso, it is unlikely that all actions or sequences will be completed correctly or with any consistency.

Note on balance

As there is considerable movement in the horizontal plane about the vertical axis, changes in the body's centre of gravity will occur in the sagittal plane, as well as in the shooting plane (see Chapter 6, Foundation Unit Analysis, p. 132).

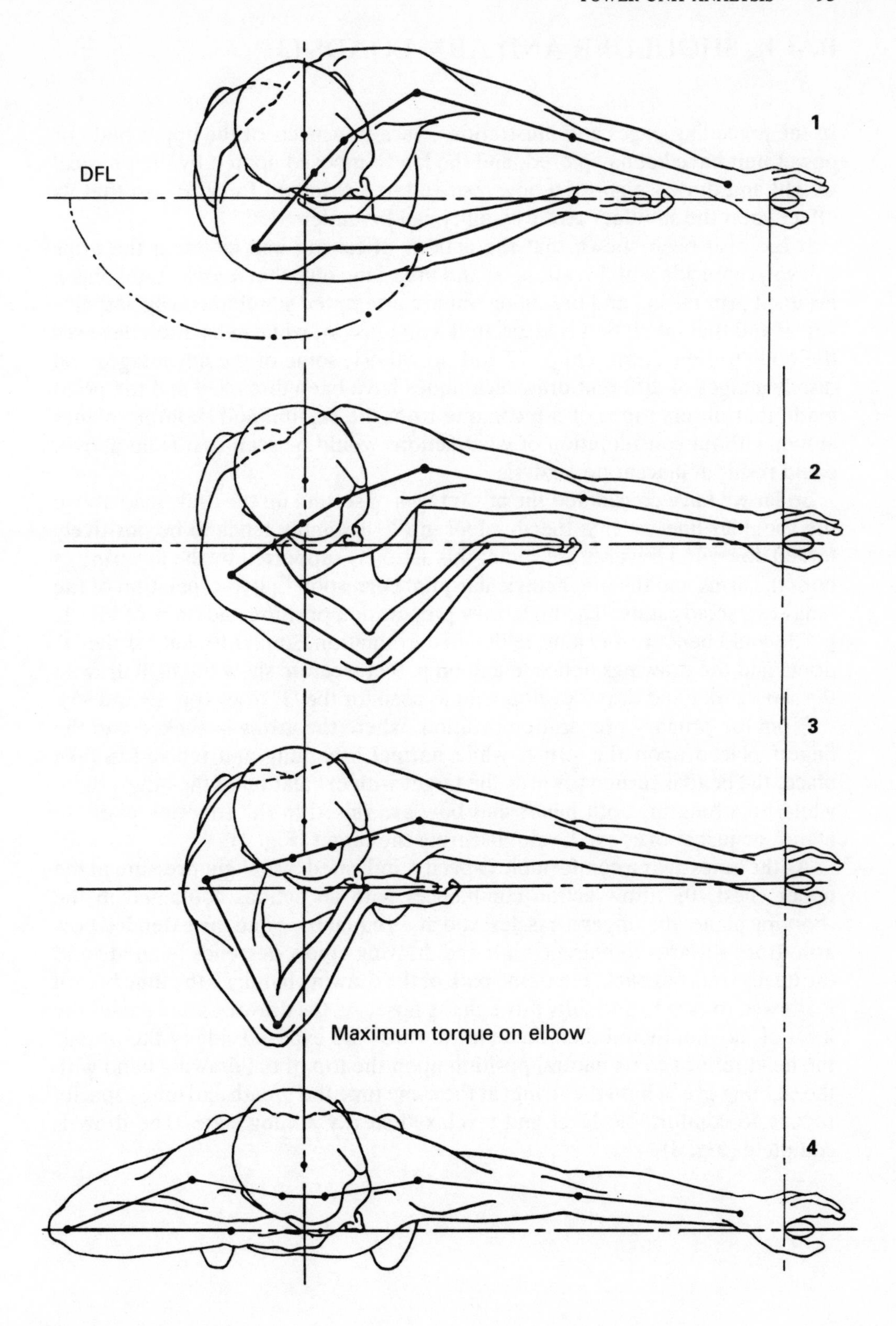
DFL
1
2
3
Maximum torque on elbow
4

BACK, SHOULDER AND ARM LOADS (3)

In the preceding pages and illustrations, various aspects of the upper body or power unit have been explored, and the loads imposed upon it by the physical weight and draw weight of a bow resolved to a resultant force 'R', so that its effect upon the shoulder girdle stability can be understood.

It has also been shown that the actions of raising and lowering the arms sideways coincide with breathing in and breathing out; that muscle antagonism occurs if arm raising and breathing out are attempted simultaneously and vice versa; and that inhalation is associated with tension, while exhalation disposes the body to relaxation. On p. 72 and pp. 90–94, some of the advantages and disadvantages of different draw techniques have been discussed and the point made that observations of a technique from the sagittal and shooting planes alone, without consideration of what actions would be seen best from above, could result in inaccurate analysis.

So far we have considered the advantages of setting up the draw load above the shoulder line, so that the shoulder girdle assembly tends to be positively forced down and towards the spine; this action is supported by the lowering of both the arms and the inner clavicular joint corresponding to exhalation of the lungs to a steady state. The high draw preparation position and draw of Fig. 1, p. 73, could benefit from a more detailed evaluation, similar to that for the 'T' draw, and the drawings opposite and on p. 99 therefore show the high draw in the same order and draw development as used for the 'T' draw (pp. 93 and 95).

From the primary preparation position, where the arrow is nocked and the fingers placed upon the string, while normal breathing and relaxation take place, the head is turned towards the target with exhalation of the lungs; then, while breathing in, both hands and bow are raised in the shooting plane to about, or just above, eye level, obscuring the target (**Fig. 1**).

As the lungs near a comfortable capacity, indicated by a slight pressure in the upper chest, the draw action commences with all actions contained in the shooting plane: the upper arms descend at an equal pace and the extended bow arm drops towards the target while the drawing elbow descends in an arc and the head is relaxed back, out of the path of the drawing hand; all the time breath is allowed to escape normally through the nose. As the drawing hand passes the level of the mouth and then the chin, towards the exposed side of the throat, the head returns to its natural position upon the top of the drawing hand with the sighting eye behind the string; at the same time the breath and lung capacity reduce to comfortable level and a relaxed steady aiming state. The draw is complete (**Fig. 4**).

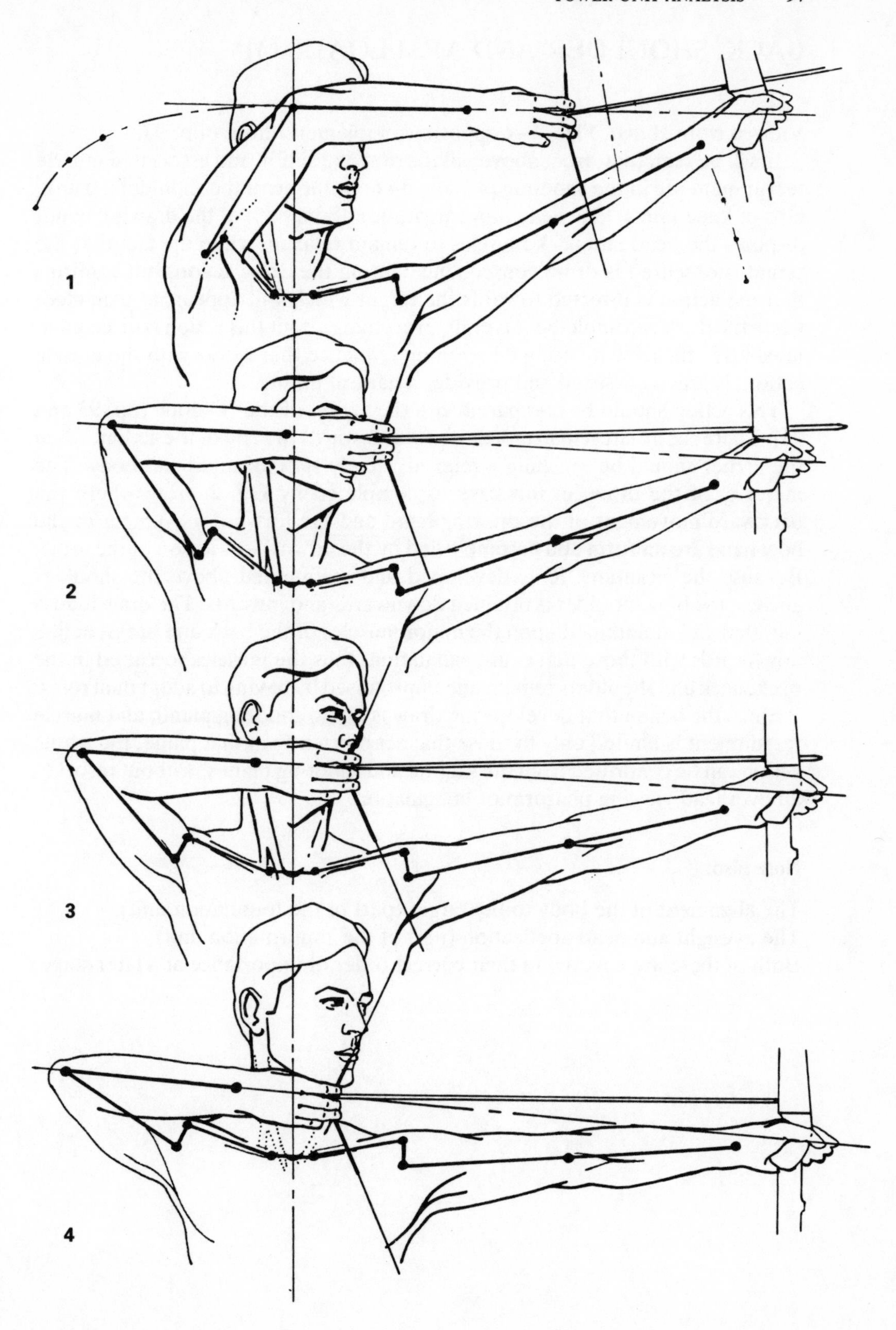
1
2
3
4

BACK, SHOULDER AND ARM LOADS (4)

Viewed from above, **Figs. 1–4** opposite complement those of p. 97.

It will be seen that, from above, all the drawing action and associated muscle recruitment are in the shooting plane, with no rotation of the shoulders, trunk, hips or knee joints. The head movement, out of the path of the drawing hand, disposes the head and neck muscles to remain relaxed, while the fact that the target is obscured is of no consequence during the draw action, but confirms that the action is directed towards the target which will appear, as expected, when the draw is completed. Overall, everything about this action is directed to maximise efficiency by using a breathing sequence that works with the muscle action, is gravity assisted and provides a natural timing.

This action should be compared with the action of the 'T' draw (pp. 93 and 95). There the greatest load and draw occur towards the end of the action, when the archer should be reaching a relaxed, steady state of mind and body. The majority of the draw, in this case, is completed by **Fig. 2**, from where the backward movement of the drawing hand and the forward movement of the bow hand are uniform and accomplished by the downwards action of the arms. Because the resultant 'R' is developed and maintained above the shoulder girdles, the bow shoulder is retained downwards and inwards. The draw load is initiated and maintained upon the major muscles of the back and breast acting downwards with those that cause exhalation; thus the muscles recruited in the back, neck and shoulders remain uncompromised by having to adopt dual roles.

Since the action that develops the draw is in the shooting plane, and muscle recruitment is limited only to those that act efficiently in that plane, the whole action can be confirmed from the sagittal and shooting planes, without resort to an overhead viewing platform or imagination.

Note also:

The alignment of the body to the target (part of the foundation unit).
The eyesight and head application (part of the confirmation unit).
Both of these are covered in their correct order of importance at a later stage.

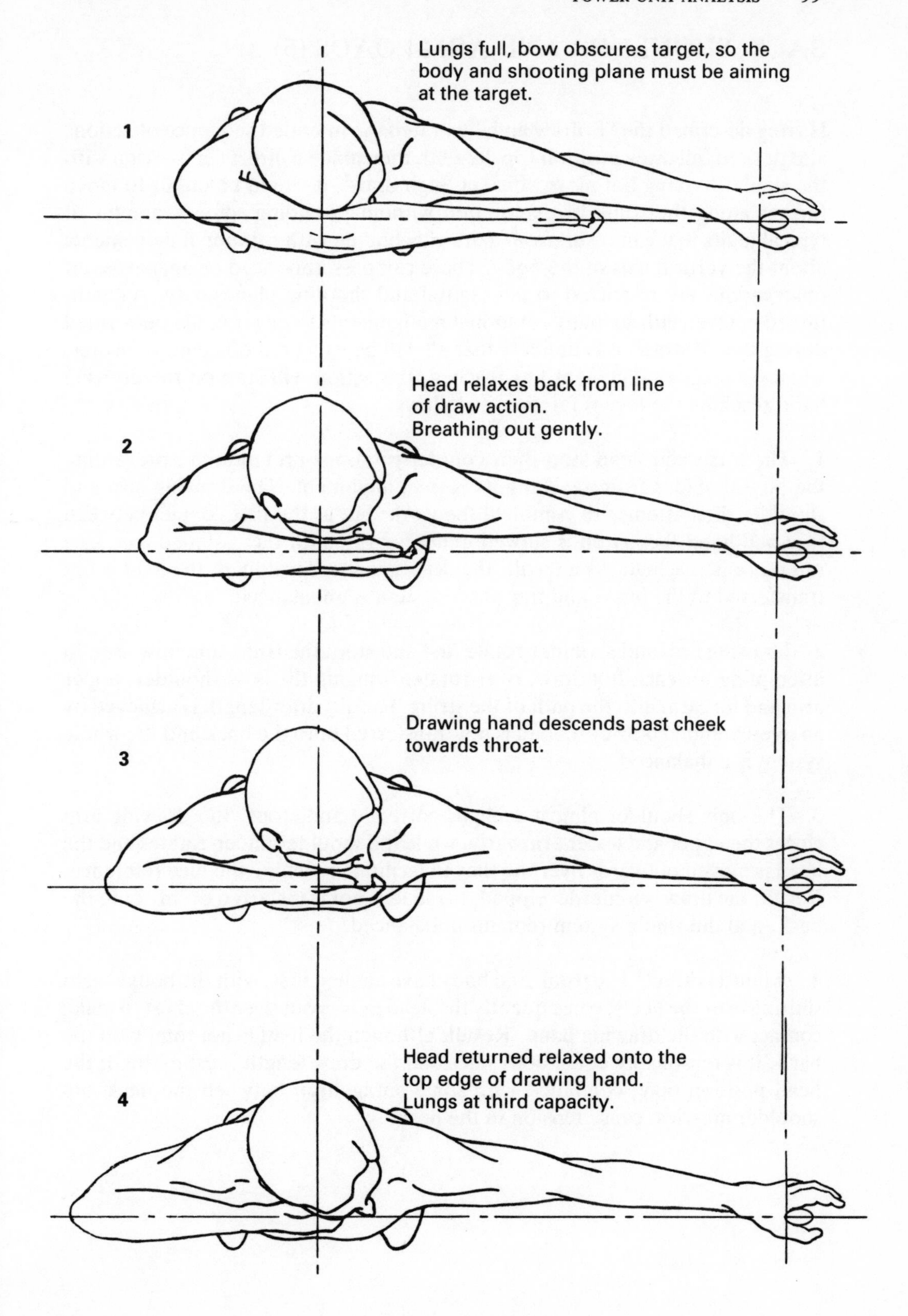
Lungs full, bow obscures target, so the body and shooting plane must be aiming at the target.
1
Head relaxes back from line of draw action.
Breathing out gently.
2
Drawing hand descends past cheek towards throat.
3
Head returned relaxed onto the top edge of drawing hand.
Lungs at third capacity.
4

BACK, SHOULDER AND ARM LOADS (5)

Having described the 'T' draw and illustrated the intended sequence of actions and desired full draw position (pp. 92–95), then made a direct comparison with the similar-looking but more efficient 'high draw', it would be unfair to move further along the route of exploration without providing some examples of typical faults that can result from a draw technique with rotational movements about the vertical axis of the body. These can pass unnoticed or unanalysed if observations are restricted to the sagittal and shooting planes only. As mentioned before, with so many rotational realignments to be correctly performed during the 'T' draw, it is unlikely that all will be executed efficiently; further, whatever stage realignment has reached, the action will stop on the drawing hand reaching the face reference, as follows:

1 The torso and head stop their counter-rotations prematurely, preventing the bow shoulder from reaching its correct alignment. The drawing arm and shoulder then attempt to complete the work, but at the first contact between face and hand the action is slowed unnecessarily until the assumed true face reference is reached. As a result, the draw is underdeveloped, the load is not transferred to the back, and the whole system is unbalanced.

2 Drawing arm and shoulder rotate first and stop; the trunk and bow arm, in attempting to reach full draw, over-rotate, bringing the bow shoulder, upper arm and forearm into the path of the string. Result: draw length is achieved by an overextended bow arm, load is not transferred onto the back and the whole system is unbalanced.

3 The bow shoulder almost realigns correctly and stops, the drawing arm closes the upper and lower arm early, while the shoulder under-rotates and the head is moved outwards over the toes to facilitate reaching the face reference. Result: the draw is underdeveloped, the load is not transferred evenly onto the back, and the whole system remains unbalanced.

4 Almost correct. The trunk and body have aligned first, with the bodyweight shifting over the heels; consequently the head moves out over the chest to make contact with the drawing hand. Result: although the load is not totally on the back, it is reasonably equal both sides and the draw length is established; the head position may, combined with some antagonism between the neck and shoulder muscles, cause tension in the neck.

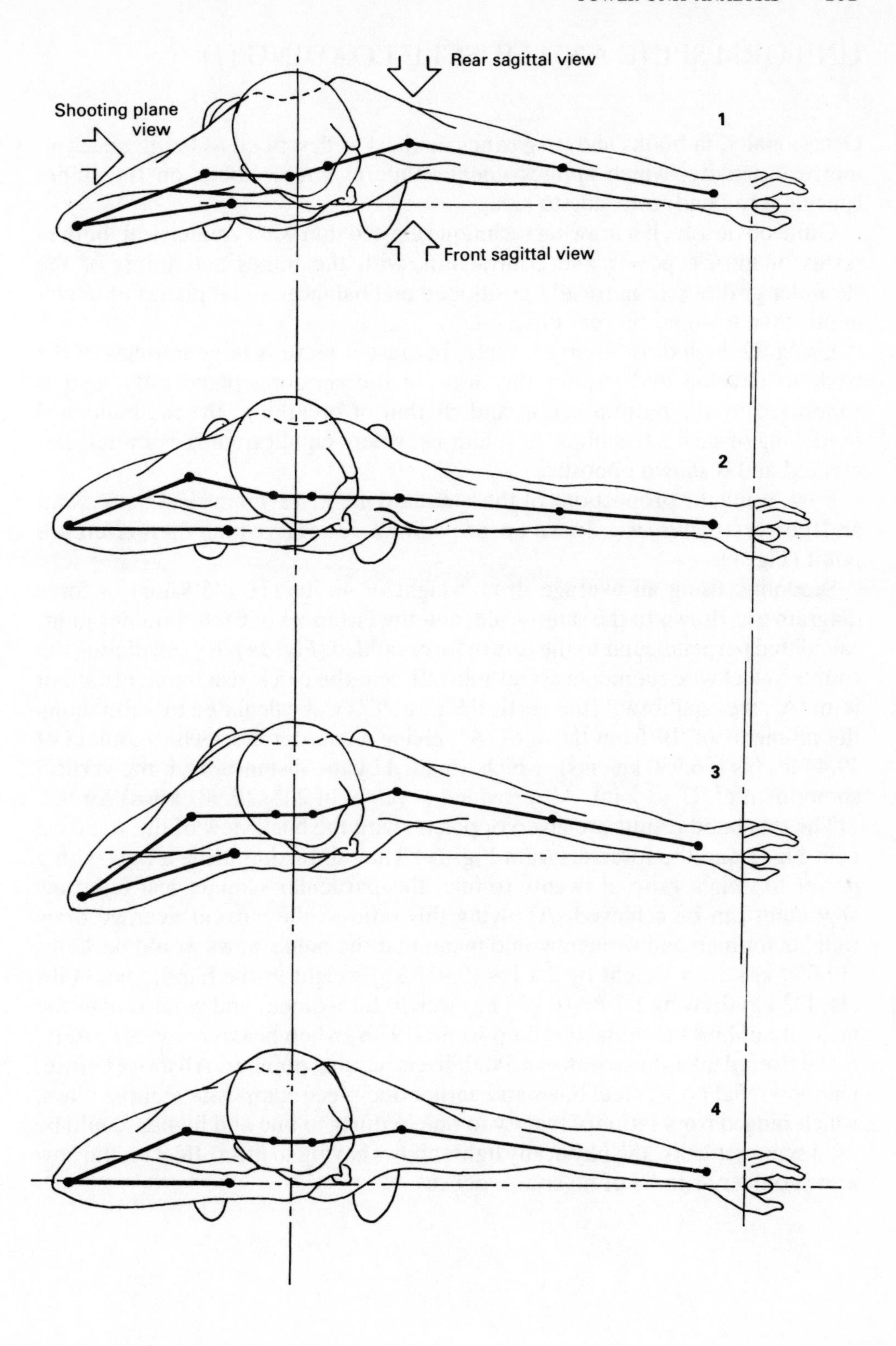
Rear sagittal view
Shooting plane view
1
Front sagittal view
2
3
4

UNIFORM SPINE AND MUSCLE LOADING (1)

Occasionally, in books and magazines, archery is described as being an asymmetrical activity, which applies unequal lateral muscle loads on the spine, causing it to bend from side to side.

Quite obviously, if a drawing technique existed that was symmetrical, both in terms of muscle power and contraction, with the bones and joints of the shoulder girdles symmetrically positioned and balanced in all planes of movement, then it would be very efficient.

Using the high draw as an example, because it recruits large muscles of the back to develop and sustain the draw in the shooting plane only, and is supported by the natural action and rhythm of breathing, the mathematical modelling of such a technique at full draw, where equilibrium is essential, was created and is shown opposite.

First, using the proportions of the 'standard man,' a symmetrical bone, joint and muscle structure was drawn up, providing a side of face under jaw reference point (**Fig. 1**).

Secondly, using an average draw weight of 40 lbs (18.145 kilos), a force diagram was drawn to the same scale, and the distances of each shoulder joint, calculated perpendicular to the line of force, added (**Fig. 1a**). By calculating the counter-clockwise moments about joint 'B' and the clockwise moments about joint 'A', the equilibrant (the vertical load at 'C') was calculated by subtracting the moments of 'B' from those of 'A', giving a counter-clockwise moment of 49.44 lbs/ins (56.950 kg/cms), which, divided by the distance from the vertical component of 'C' to joint 'A', provided a weight of 2 lbs (0.907 kilos) for 'C'.

The tabulated results are given opposite, with the back view of the standard man **Fig. 1** and the force diagram **Fig. 1a**. They show that using a bow with a power to weight ratio of twenty to one, this particular symmetrical full draw alignment can be achieved. Applying this ratio to the current average draw weights for men and women would mean that the men's bows would be 42 lbs (19.050 kg) draw weight by 2.1 lbs (0.952 kg) weight in the hand, and 34 lbs (15.422 kg) draw by 1.7 lbs (0.453 kg) weight for women, and would cover the majority of bows manufactured up to the 1970s, when heavier wooden risers, metal risered take-down bows and stabilisers became popular. All those before, longbows, flat bows, steel bows and earlier one-piece composite recurve bows, which ranged from ratios of twenty to one to thirty to one and higher, could be used symmetrically, the physically lighter bows having so little effect on the bow arm shoulder as to be of no consequence.

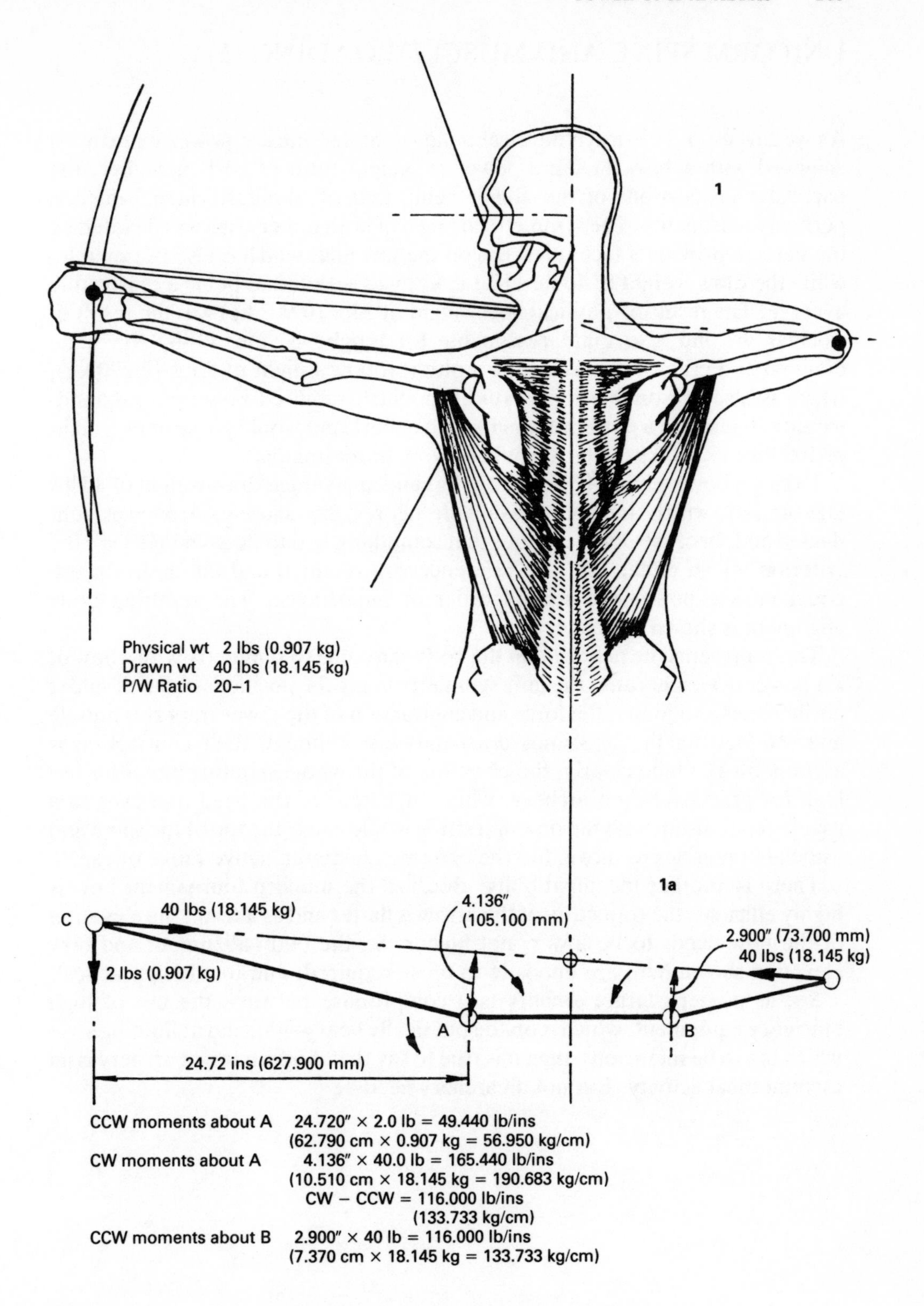

CCW moments about A 24.720″ × 2.0 lb = 49.440 lb/ins
(62.790 cm × 0.907 kg = 56.950 kg/cm)
CW moments about A 4.136″ × 40.0 lb = 165.440 lb/ins
(10.510 cm × 18.145 kg = 190.683 kg/cm)
CW − CCW = 116.000 lb/ins
(133.733 kg/cm)
CCW moments about B 2.900″ × 40 lb = 116.000 lb/ins
(7.370 cm × 18.145 kg = 133.733 kg/cm)

UNIFORM SPINE AND MUSCLE LOADING (2)

As we saw on p. 103, a symmetrical bone, joint and muscle power unit can be achieved with a bow having a power to weight ratio of 20:1 or higher, the particular proportions of the archer being that of 'standard' man, which is perfectly reasonable. The symmetrical angle of both upper arms was dictated by the need to provide a face reference on the jaw line, which is also reasonable, while the draw weight of 40 lbs (18.145 kg) was selected as being a reasonable average. The resulting physical bow weight of 2 lbs (0.907 kg) was the result of calculation, and also quite reasonable for longbows, etc. Using the same diagram and criteria, but selecting a physical bow weight of 5 lbs (2.270 kg), which is also reasonable for a typical modern stabilised bow or compound, would still result in a power to weight ratio of 20:1, but would give a draw weight of 100 lbs (45.360 kg), which would be very unreasonable.

Taking a bow weight of 5 lbs (2.270 kg) and an average draw weight of 40 lbs (18.145 kg), which are both reasonable figures, the same exercise was conducted and, because it was obvious that something had to be asymmetrical, the criterion for an under-jaw face reference was retained and the desire to use equal muscle power the second order of importance. The resulting body alignment is shown opposite.

This represents the nearest that the body can come to symmetry with a bow of 8:1 power to weight ratio, the only symmetry being the positions of the shoulder girdle bones and joints, the force and contraction of the lower trapezius muscle and the load on the latissimus dorsi muscles, although their contraction is asymmetrical. Quite clearly, the elevation of the whole shooting unit is far too high for practical target archery, while alignment of the head and eyes to a usable relationship with the bow and string would cause the top of the spine and associated muscles to move into the extreme maximum active range of use.

There is another incompatibility. Because the modern tournament bow is highly efficient, the trajectory of the arrow is flatter and as a result the elevation of the bow needs to be lower, not higher. So the body alignment and bow elevation shown here are opposite to those required, and totally impractical.

So, as modern target archery is a compromise between the use of high efficiency equipment, which is on the physically heavy side, and a shooting style which has to be inefficient, then it is true to say that modern target archery is an asymmetrical activity. But not all archery need be.

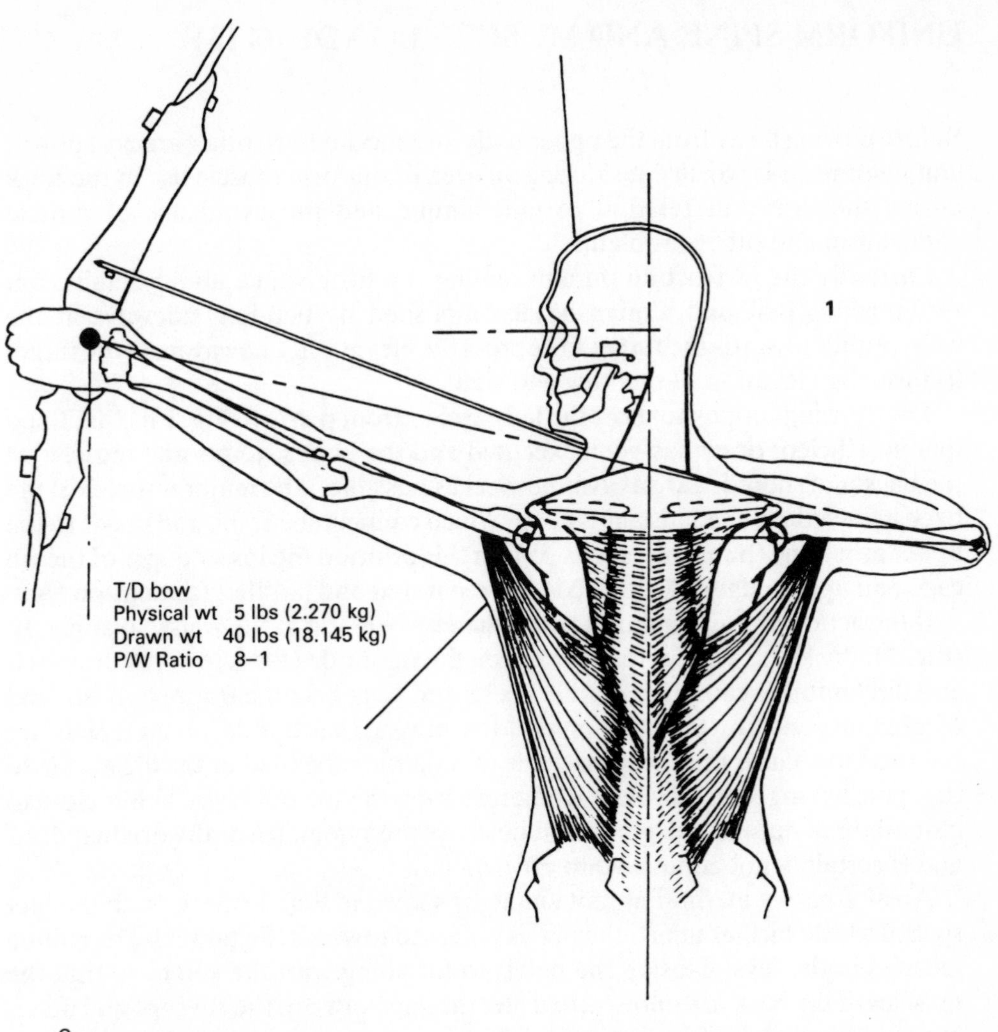

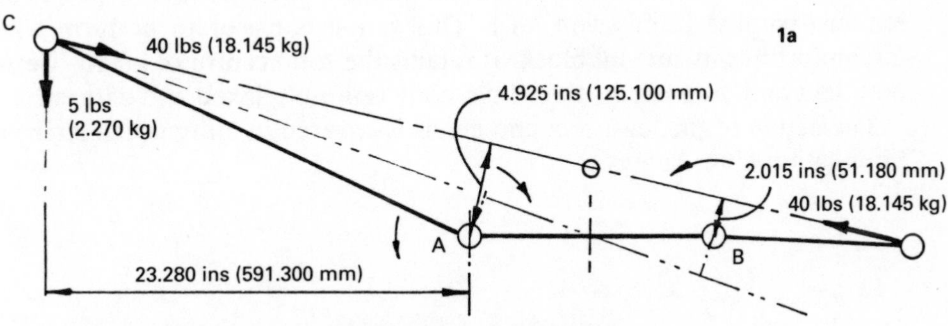

CCW moments about A	23.800″ × 5.0 lb = 116.400 lb/ins
	(59.130 cm × 2.270 kg = 134.230 kg/cm)
CW moments about A	4.925″ × 40.0 lb = 197.000 lb/ins
	(12.510 cm × 18.145 kg = 227.000 kg/cm approx)
	CW − CCW = 80.600 lb/ins
	(92.800 kg/cm)
CCW moments about B	2.015″ × 40.0 lb = 80.600 lb/ins
	(5.118 cm × 18.145 kg = 92.800 kg/cm approx)

UNIFORM SPINE AND MUSCLE LOADING (3)

Before moving away from the upper body and shoulders to other areas of power unit analysis, it is worth considering an area of uniform muscle use in the back during the draw, in relation to unit aiming and the avoidance of muscle antagonism and other problems.

Currently the instruction on unit aiming is a little vague about details, but recommends that unit aiming be accomplished by bending sideways at the waist, either towards the target to depress the elevation, or away from the target to raise the elevation of the bow and sight.

The drawings opposite show the lady archer from p. 67. In **Fig. 1** it is assumed that an efficient draw has been executed and the bones, joints and muscles of the back and shoulder are as symmetrical as possible. The major muscles of the back involved are the latissimus dorsi, which connect the spine and pelvis to the upper arm bone (humerus, see p. 35). In this position the lower edges of the rib cage and upper edges of the pelvis are separated and parallel (dimension 'A').

If the action of unit aiming is performed by bending at the waist, to angle 'B' (**Fig. 2**), the lower edge of the rib cage on the right side closes towards the pelvis and discomfort is caused as clothes, belts and flesh become trapped. Also, and of greater concern, the latissimus dorsi muscles each side of the spine are required to change their lengths while maintaining the load of the draw, due to the spine having to bend where it emerges from the top of pelvis. This is close to a situation of muscle antagonism; it destroys the symmetry of the original draw and is certainly not conducive to efficiency.

An alternative method of unit aiming is shown in **Fig. 3** where, with the feet spaced a little farther apart, the pelvis is moved towards the target by recruiting muscles in the legs, causing the pelvis to tilt along with the spine, so that the muscles of the back are undisturbed and the gap between the rib cage and pelvis remains parallel (dimension 'A'). This action is easier to perform without discomfort or any mental block; it retains the total centre of gravity between both feet and, as a result, the whole body is more relaxed and natural.

The action of the legs, feet and pelvis is covered in more detail later under Foundation Unit Analysis.

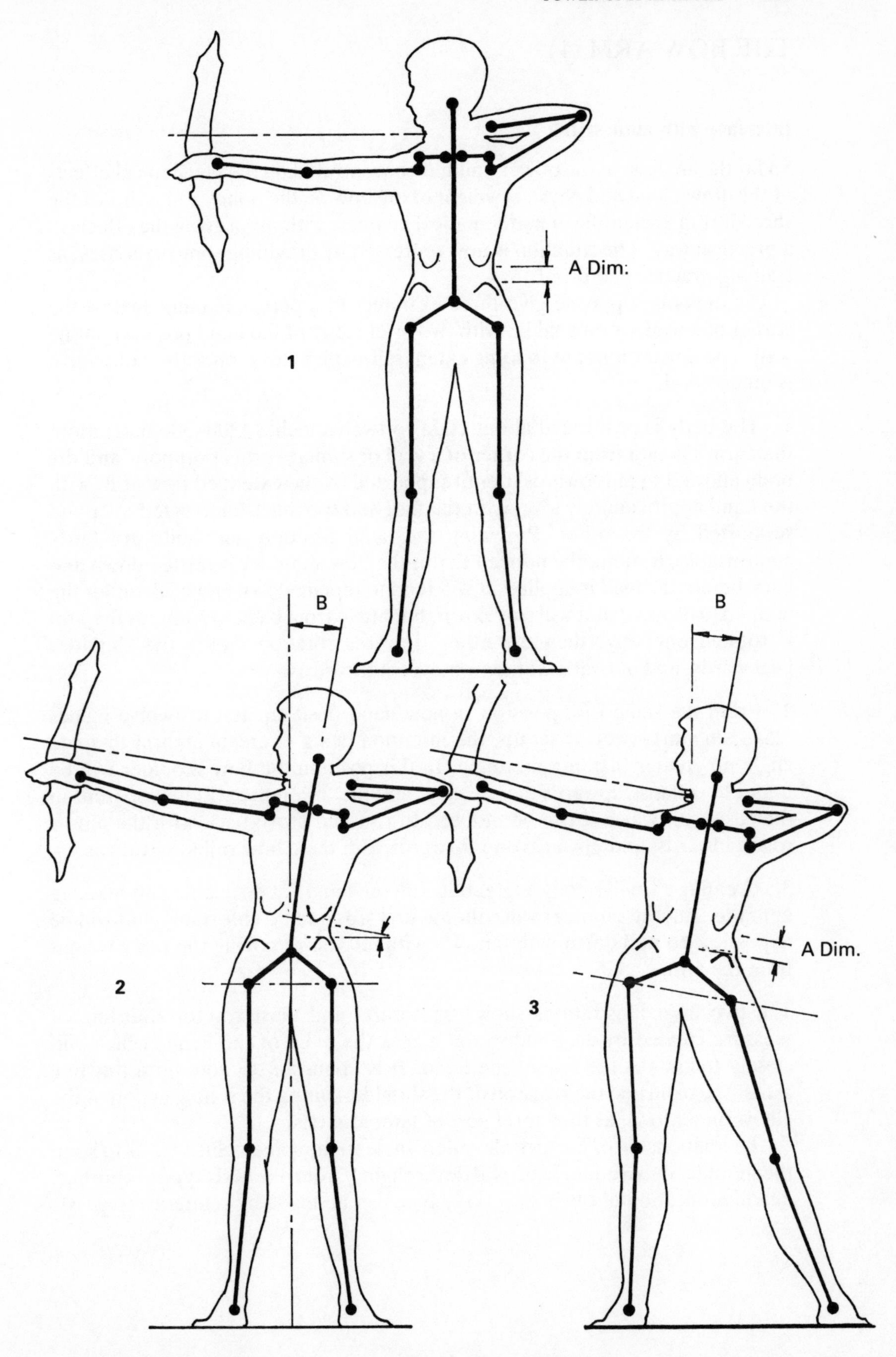
A Dim:
1
B
B
2
A Dim.
3

THE BOW ARM (1)

Interface with main trunk

So far the analysis of the power unit has concentrated on the mechanical effects of the drawn load and physical weight of the bow on the bones and joints of the shoulders in a scientific or mathematical manner, without proving the effects in a practical way. The situation is now redressed by providing some exercises, as training practice and proof.

The drawings opposite give three examples of a person leaning against the corner of a wall, or on a table, with two inset views of the hand position on the wall. The illustrations are to some extent self-explanatory, once their objective is understood.

1 The body is positioned about eight to twelve inches (200–306 mm) more than arm's length from the corner of a wall or similar vertical support, and the body allowed to fall towards it until supported by the extended bow arm, with the hand approximately level with the face and the inner leg crossed over and supported by the other. Providing the hand position and body are fairly comfortable, it should be noticed that if the bow shoulder is settled down and back before the load is applied, it will tend to remain down and back under the applied load and that it will stay down, but move from back to front, as the arm is rotated one way, then the other. Inwards rotation moves the shoulder backwards, and outwards rotation moves it forwards.

2 From the same foot position, a new hand position, ten to twelve inches (254–306 mm) lower, is set up, the intention being to create an arm-to-spine angle no greater than a right angle. In this position the bow shoulder will be found to collapse upwards more easily, and the difference will be apparent in the ease with which it can be induced to rise and move back with the elbow rolled inwards, and upwards and forwards with the elbow rolled outwards.

3 Creating a similar body angle, but with the hand flat on a table and relaxing onto the arm, the shoulder will collapse upwards quite comfortably, but will be impossible to pull down with muscles without first removing the body weight from the arm.

The two inset illustrations show the natural and most comfortable line of pressure created by each individual across the palm of the hand, which will closely follow the life line of the hand. It is important to note both this line across the palm and the reaction of the shoulder during the rolling action of the elbow under load, as they form part of later analysis.

The relationship of the arm elevation angle to the spine, which tends to keep the shoulder down under load, will differ slightly from one body type to another, and identification of one's own body type can be made by reference to p. 81.

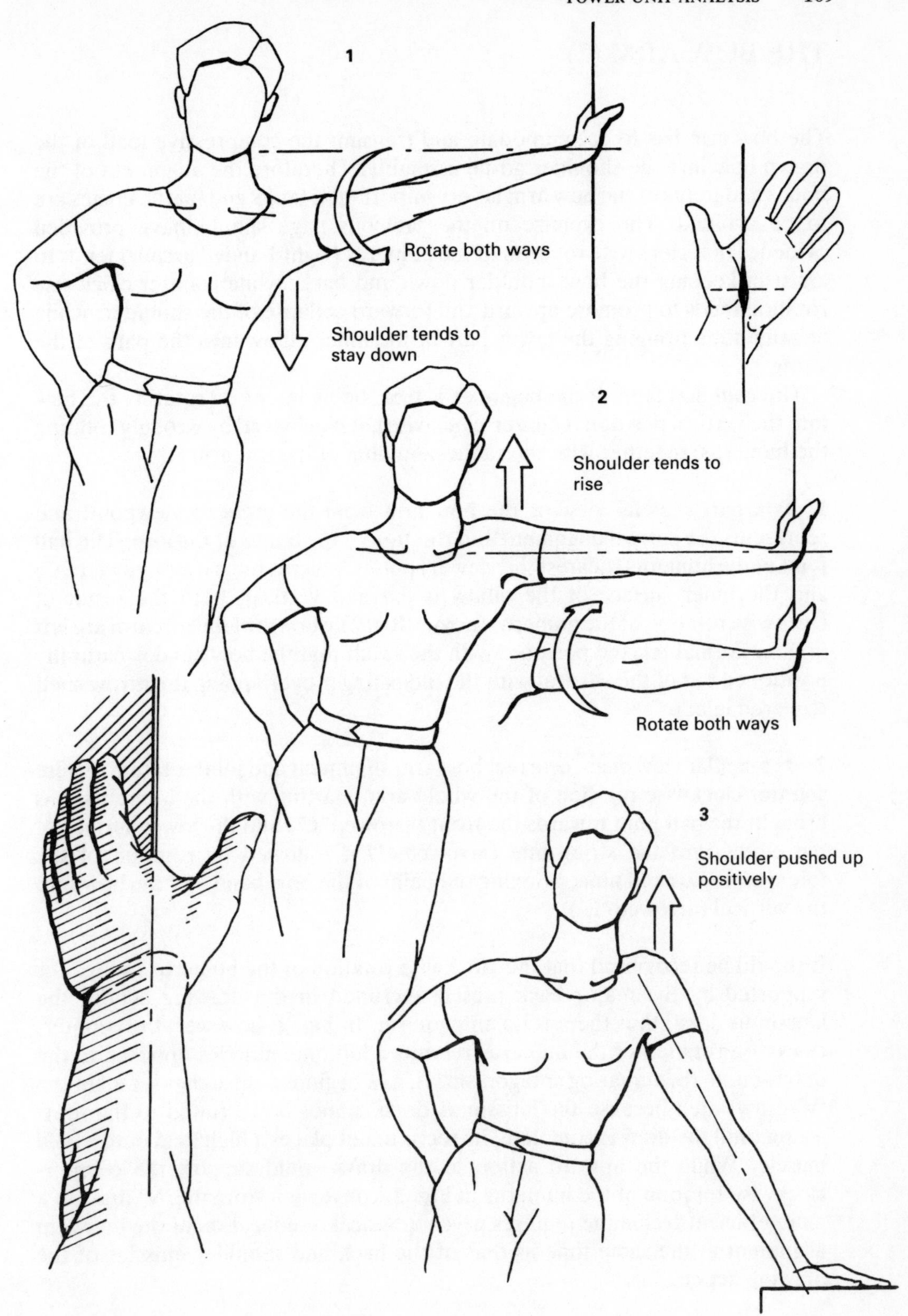
1
Rotate both ways
Shoulder tends to stay down
2
Shoulder tends to rise
Rotate both ways
3
Shoulder pushed up positively

THE BOW ARM (2)

The bow arm has to accommodate and transmit the compressive load of the drawn bow into the shoulder girdle assembly. Therefore the alignment of the bones and joints of the bow arm is very important if faults and inefficiencies are to be avoided. The exercise on the previous page should have provided evidence that clockwise rotation of the humerus (right-handed archer) tends to assist in keeping the bow shoulder down and back, while counter-clockwise rotation tends to promote upward and forward collapse of the shoulder, while at same time bringing the lower part of the inner elbow into the path of the string.

The common fault of the beginner is that, being intent on rotating the bow into the vertical position (counter-clockwise), it is achieved by wrongly rotating the humerus, together with the radius and ulna of the forearm.

1 Is a part skeletal view of the bow arm from the archer's viewpoint and represents the correct alignment and rotation of the bones of the arm. The ball joint of the humerus (nearest the viewer) points towards the back (arrowed 'A') and the inner surface of the elbow is flat and vertical, both the result of clockwise rotation of the humerus (arrow 'B'). The bones of the forearm are left in their normal relaxed position, with the result that the bow hand is naturally positioned out of the vertical with the index finger overlapping the arrow shelf (covered later).

2 Is a similar view of an incorrect bow arm alignment and joint rotation, where counter-clockwise rotation of the whole arm, starting with the humerus, has brought the ball joint towards the front (arrowed 'C') and the lower surface of the elbow into the string line (arrowed 'D'), followed by rotation of the forearm, radius and ulna, bringing the palm of the bow hand and the bow into the vertical (arrowed 'E').

It should be recognised that the clockwise rotation of the humerus in **Fig. 1** is supported by the major back muscle recruited in the drawing action, the latissimus dorsi; thus there is no antagonism. In **Fig. 2**, however, the counter-clockwise rotation of the humerus recruits additional muscles opposed to the draw action, thus creating antagonism. If, as a beginner, an archer is taught the 'V' draw, then because the latissimus dorsi cannot be recruited to the draw action until the draw is complete, its recruitment places a high load onto a cold muscle. While the upward action of the draw would support the counter-clockwise rotation of the humerus in **Fig. 2**, conversion from the 'V' draw to a more efficient technique requires psychophysical re-education of the bow arm alignment at the same time as that of the back and shoulder muscles of the drawing action.

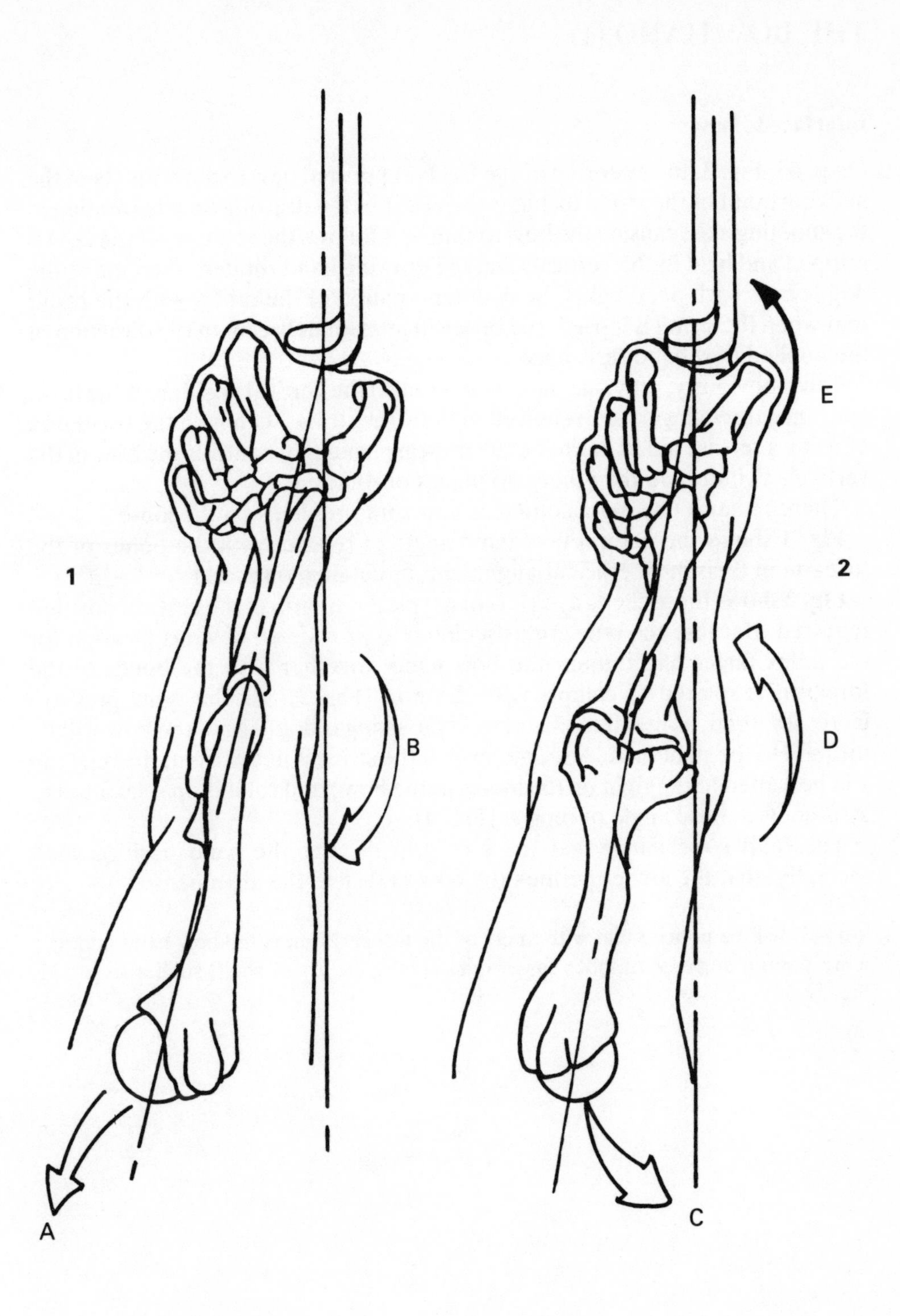
1
2
A
B
C
D
E

THE BOW HAND (1)

Interface to bow

On p. 55, Fig. 3, the castoring of the freely supported bow to movements of the nocking point of the string includes the effect of the drawing fingers rotating in the shooting axis, causing the bow to cant as it follows the rotation. If the bow is gripped and held in the vertical, and the drawing hand rotated, then the string dog-legs as each hand fights the counter-rotation of the other, with the result that when the string is loosed, the bow will immediately cant in the direction of the applied bow hand resistance.

Quite obviously, only one hand must control the vertical position of the bow, and since three fingers are required to draw the string, then with the exception of using a release aid, it has to be the drawing hand that controls the bow in the vertical, as it does in the other two planes of rotation.

There remains one more source of bow cant problems on the loose.

Fig. 1 shows the natural bow hand angle of repose, with the bones of the forearm in their most efficient alignment, as detailed on p. 111.

Fig. 2 shows the archer's eye view of a typical bow grip in the vertical position required. Because the bow grip is sculpted to provide an obvious location for the index finger and thumb, the bow hand, together with the bones of the forearm, is rotated to comply with the grip (**Fig. 3**). As the draw pressure increases, then, as mentioned above, if the string is dog-legged the bow will be torqued to the right on release, but even if the string is not twisted, the bow can still be canted to the right on the loose, as the bow hand rotates on relaxation to assume its natural angle of repose (**Fig. 4**).

The fault is primarily that the bow grip dictates the hand position and, secondly, that the archer permits the bow to dictate the alignment.

NOTE: It will be noticed that with many of the top performers the bow hand adopts a more natural angle, with index finger overlapping the arrow shelf, similar to p. 111, Fig. 1.

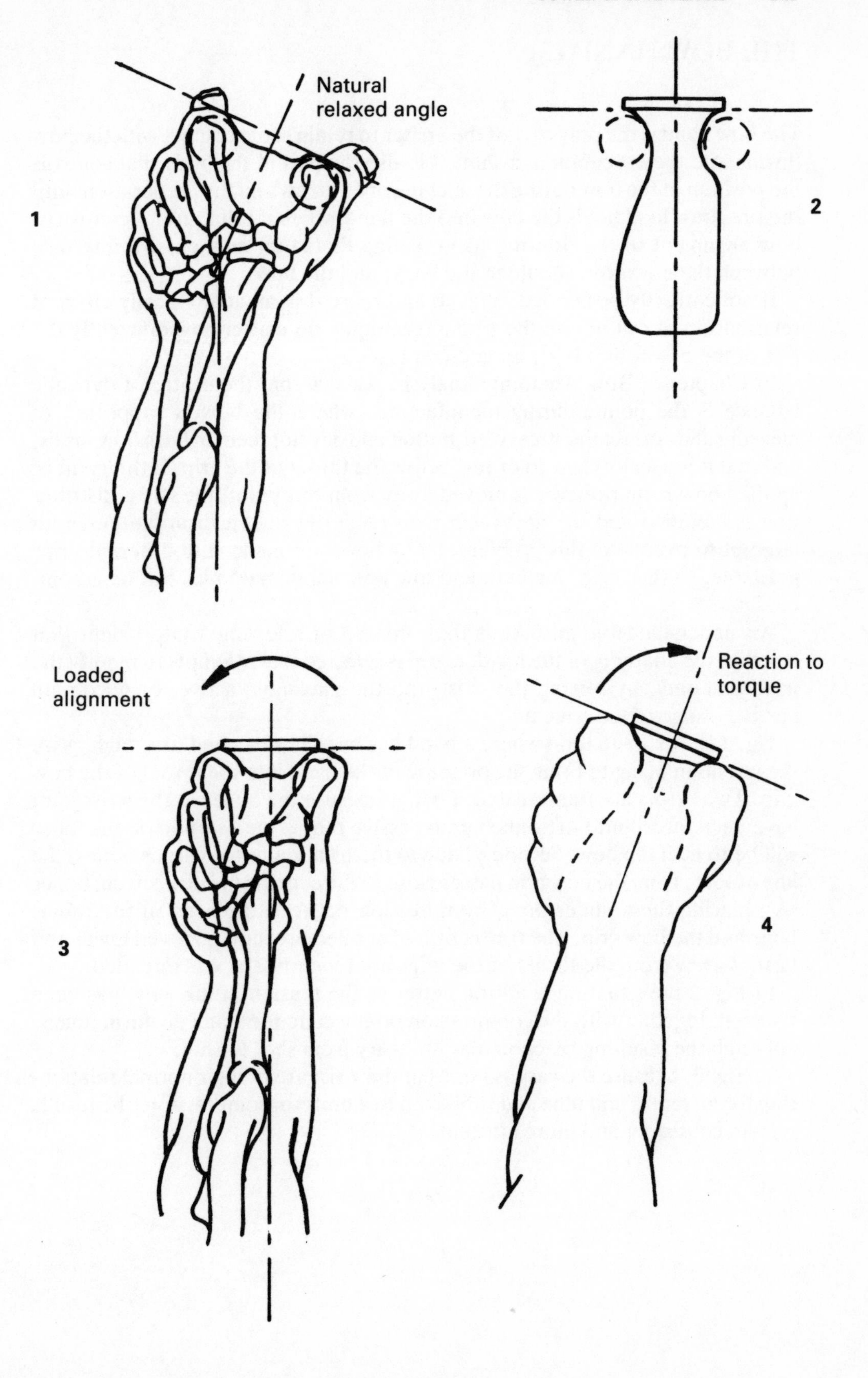
Natural
relaxed angle
1
2
Loaded
alignment
3
Reaction to
torque
4

THE BOW HAND (2)

The bow hand is the only part of the archer to retain some contact with the bow throughout the execution of a shot. It is also the part of the body that controls the position of the bow during the nocking of an arrow and the preparation until the pre-draw load holds the bow into the hand, when it relinquishes control of bow alignment to the drawing hand, acting thereafter as a passive interface between the bow arm, shoulder and back, and the bow.

If not correctly positioned, aligned and relaxed in an anatomically efficient relationship, it can negate the whole technique, no matter how efficiently the rest of the power unit is set up and employed.

In Chapter 3, Bow Anatomy Analysis, we saw that the centre of dynamic balance is the point, during manufacture, where the bow is supported to measure and correct the stress distribution and development in both bow limbs, and that it is usually close to or just below the throat of the grip. If the point of applied bow hand pressure is moved away from this point, the stress distribution is modified and the limbs will then react out of synchronisation. In an attempt to overcome this problem, many bows are made with different grips available, so that high, medium and low bow hand anatomies can be accommodated.

An understandable mistake is that, instead of selecting a grip height that matches the anatomy of the hand, a grip is selected that attempts to modify the hand anatomy, by forcing the wrist into the maximum active, or maximum passive, range of movement.

Fig. 1 shows a situation where a hand has been mismatched to a 'high' grip, the intention being to bring the pressure of the hand into the throat of the bow grip. Two errors are thus created, Firstly, because the bones of the wrist joint have been forced into their maximum passive range, the reaction on the loose will be to heel the bow. Secondly, due to the rotation of the carpus bones, the line of force from the bow arm passes close to the cuneiform and pisiform bones 'A', placing them under direct compression between the head of the radius bone and the bow grip. The true centre of applied pressure is moved lower and farther away from the throat of the grip, not towards it as was intended.

In **Fig. 2** the situation is a little better as the tension in the wrist has been reduced, together with the compression on the cuneiform and pisiform bones, although the resulting reaction may still vary from shot to shot.

In **Fig. 3**, because the carpus bones of the wrist are in their normal relationship to the radius and ulna and subjected to a uniform compression, the results remain consistent and more efficient.

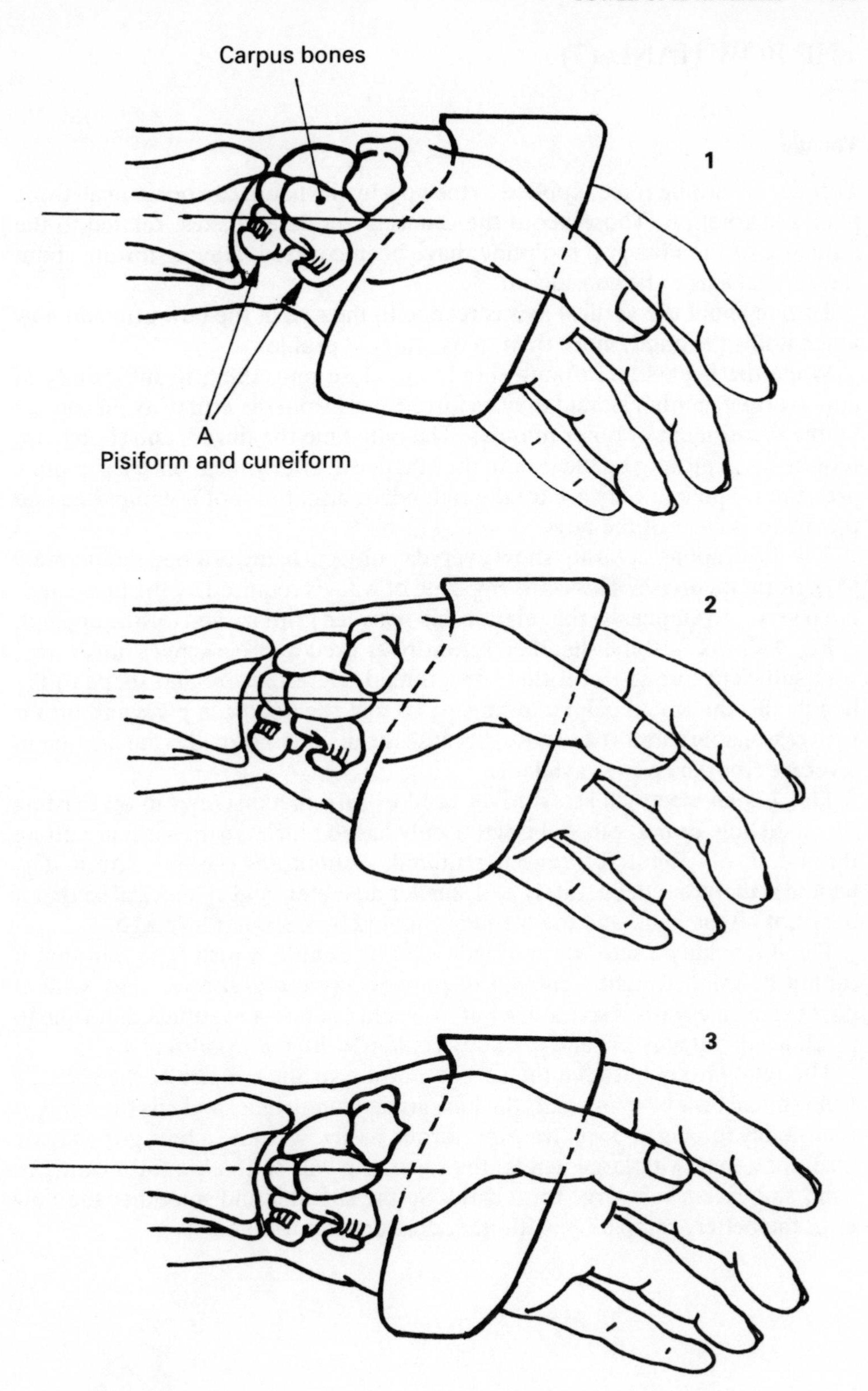
Carpus bones
1
A
Pisiform and cuneiform
2
3

THE BOW HAND (3)

Torque

Torque, or turning force, applied to the bow by the hand, can occur in all three planes of rotation. Those about the shooting and lateral axes, related to the influence of the bow grip sculpting, have been covered, leaving torque about the vertical axis to be considered.

Torque about the vertical axis is related to the size of the bow grip and how much it fills the hand, more than to its sculpted profile.

While the fingers and thumb should not close onto the grip sufficiently to apply torque, neither should they be forced away from the grip to avoid contact by the recruitment of other muscles. The only time the fingers and thumb are required is in picking up the bow in the first place, after which, once a pre-draw pressure is applied, they are totally redundant until the shot is completed and the arrow is clear of the bow.

The illustrations opposite show everyday objects being gripped deliberately to perform their task. This is the opposite of what is required by the bow hand, but it serves to emphasise the relationship between grip size and torque applied.

Fig. 1 shows a cabinet-handled screwdriver used to drive screws into wood, with sufficient torque to cut their own thread. Here the size and shape of the handle fills the whole palm and fingers, so that the hand can push and turn it with reasonable comfort and ease, because the diameter provides the maximum leverage from the power available.

Fig. 2 is an electrical screwdriver used to turn metal screws in an existing threaded hole or nut. Since the screw only has to pinch a wire without cutting through it, only limited torque is required, without any pushing action. The handle is therefore deliberately of a smaller diameter, and cylindrical so that it does not fill the hand and the torque is limited by a smaller leverage.

Fig. 3 is simply a screwdriver blade with no handle, which is so thin that it cannot be gripped tightly enough to provide any useful torque, and while it might spin an electrical screw in a nut, it would not transmit sufficient torque to pinch a wire effectively, and certainly could not drive a wood screw.

The relationship between the size of a bow grip and the size of the archer's hand should now be obvious. If the bow grip is comfortable and fills the hand, it is probably too big and will transmit torque easily, so while a bow grip may be ideal for a man with large hands, the same grip will be too big for a woman's hand and excessively large for a child. So the slimmer and smoother the bow grip, the better, compatible with not being uncomfortable.

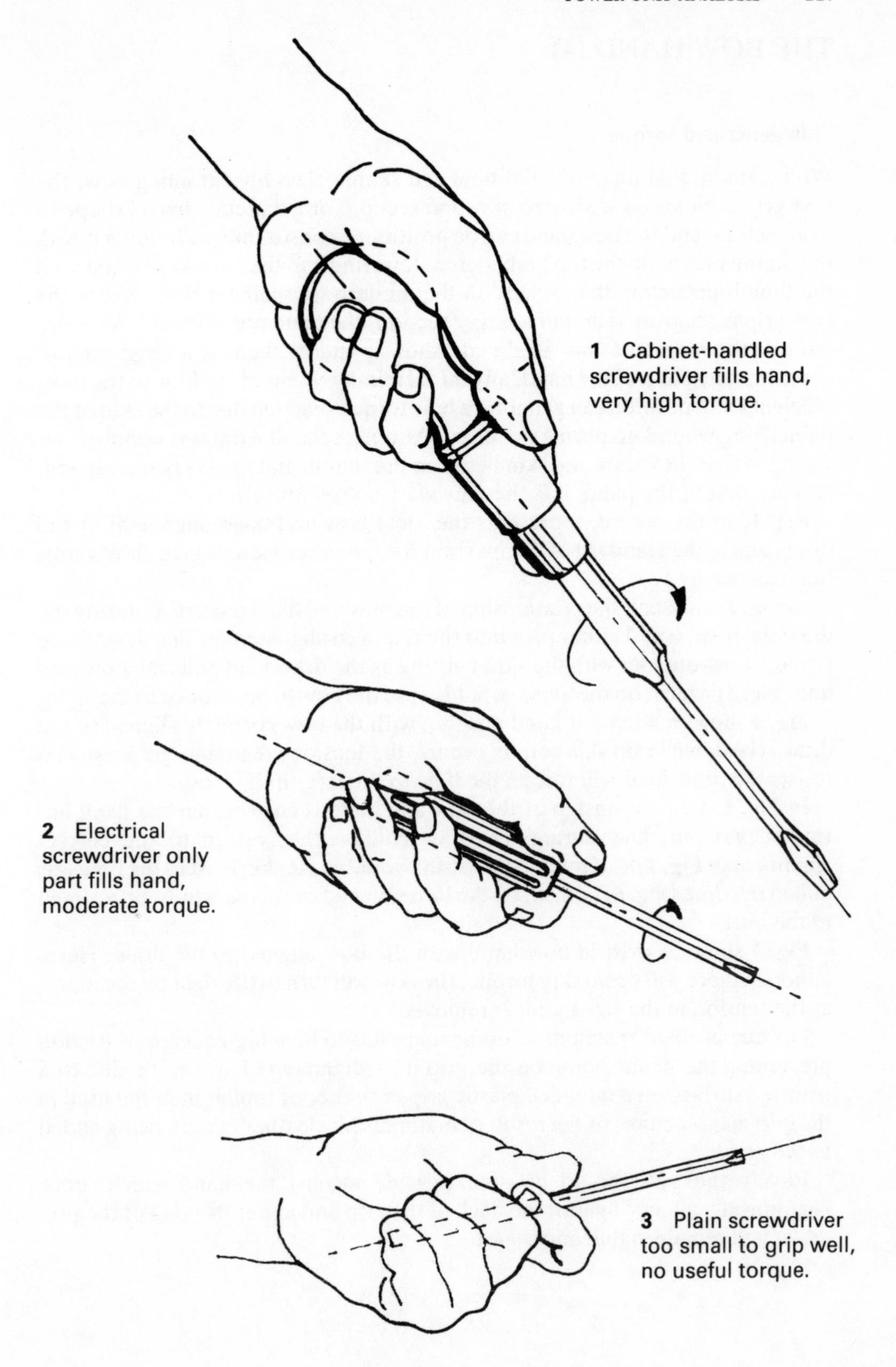
1 Cabinet-handled screwdriver fills hand, very high torque.
2 Electrical screwdriver only part fills hand, moderate torque.
3 Plain screwdriver too small to grip well, no useful torque.

THE BOW HAND (4)

Skin generated torque

With a traditional longbow, flat bow and simple glass fibre training bow, the bow grip is either cigar-shaped of round section, or a flattened barrel shape of oval section, and the bow hand can be positioned consistently by holding it with the thumb placed up the top limb, before lowering it to the normal position with the thumb encircling the grip. With the modern tournament bow, where the bow grip is sculptured and of a larger section, the hand positioning is far more critical, for many reasons as already shown, and as there is a large area of contact in the palm of the hand, any initial misalignment of the bow to the most efficient hand position can generate a bow torque reaction due to the skin of the palm being wound up during the draw. Although the illustrations opposite are wrong in that they show the skin between the thumb and fingers being twisted, and not that of the palm, it is the only way to show the effect.

Fig. 1, in the centre, represents the ideal bow and hand alignment at full draw, and is the standard of comparison for the other views which show faults that can occur.

In **Fig. 2**, although the relationship of the bow and hand is correct, during the draw the hand could either turn into the required alignment of **Fig. 1**, or could remain wrist-out and with the skin twisting as the draw load pulls the bow into line (**Fig. 3**) which, on the loose, would cause the bow to be torqued to the right.

Fig. 4 shows a wrist-out hand position with the bow correctly aligned to the draw. Here, while no skin torque occurs, the tension created in the wrist as it resists the draw load will torque the bow to the left on the loose.

In **Fig. 5** the relationship of the bow and hand is correct, but the hand has rotated wrist-in, and during the draw could either return to the correct alignment of **Fig. 1** or, if retained wrist-in, would cause skin twist as the bow was pulled into line (**Fig. 6**), which, on the loose, would cause the bow to be torqued to the left.

Fig. 7 shows a wrist-in bow hand with the bow aligned to the draw. Here, although there will be no skin torque, the bow will turn to the right on the loose, as the tension in the wrist joint is removed.

For any of these reactions to occur there has to be a high degree of friction preventing the hand sliding on the grip into alignment. This can be due to a textured surface on a moulded plastic grip, a rubber or similar material used in the grip manufacture, or the result of materials like leather or cork being added to the grip.

Ideally the grip should be able to slide against the hand which, once anatomically aligned against the back of the grip and under the load of the pre-draw, will remain stable and secure.

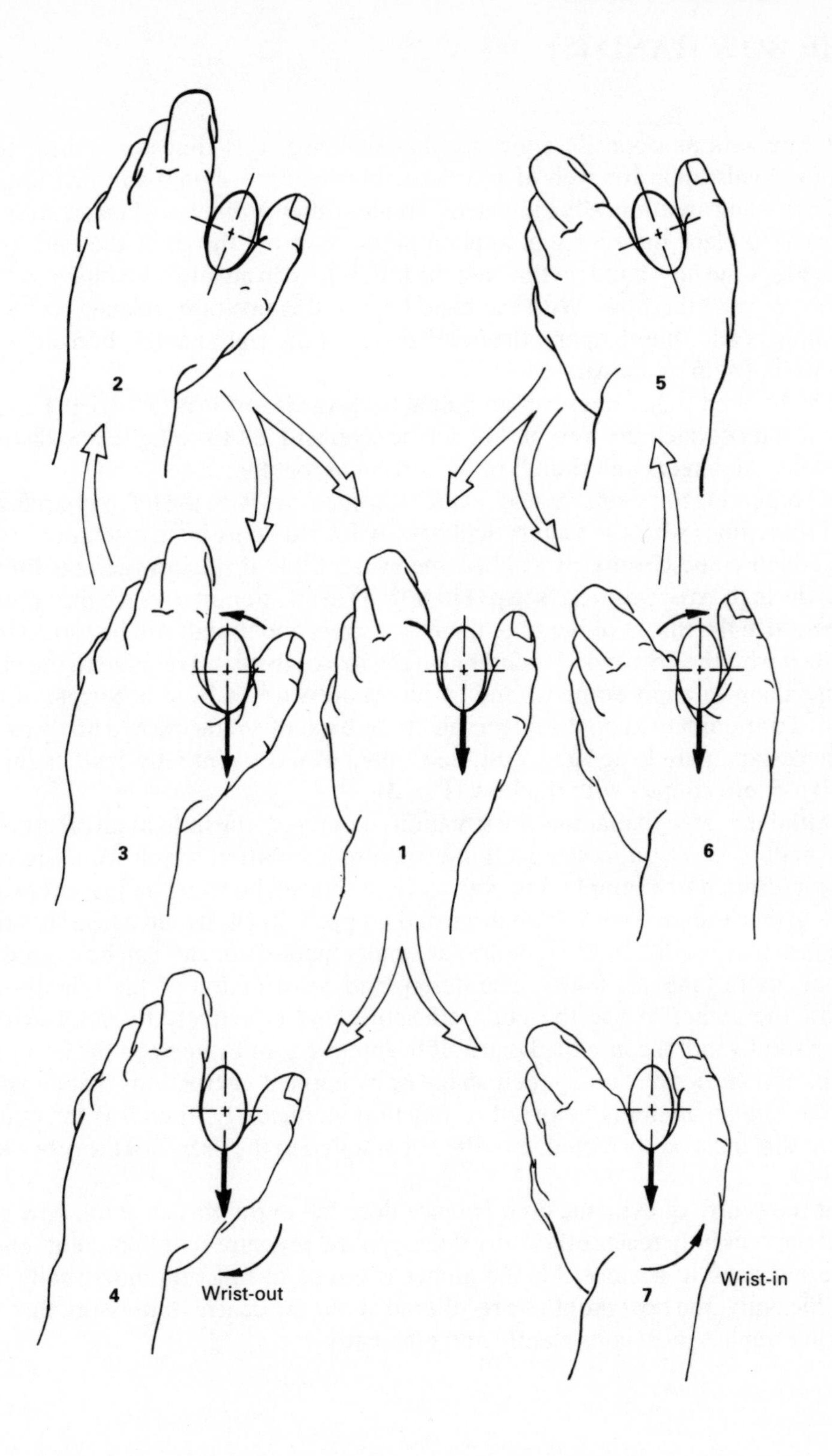
2
5
3
1
6
4
Wrist-out
7
Wrist-in

THE BOW HAND (5)

The illustrations opposite show another exercise, this time to confirm that putting loads upon the web of soft tissue between the thumb and first finger, besides being anatomically inefficient, creates other problems when an attempt is made to place the centre of applied pressure in the throat of the bow grip.

In **Fig. 1** the bow hand, in this case the left, is held in an attitude similar to that for supporting the bow. With the hand kept in this position, relaxed and with the fingers and thumb apart, the index finger of the right hand is hooked over the web of skin as shown.

The hooked right finger is then pulled backwards towards the wrist (**Fig. 2**), as a result of which the web of skin will be seen and felt to collapse and distort, drawing the fingers and thumb of the left hand together.

By repeating this exercise several times, sometimes with the left hand relaxed and sometimes with the fingers deliberately forced apart in an attempt to stop the collapse and closure, it will become evident that if the bow hand is forced into the high-wrist position (see p. 115, Fig. 1) in an attempt to place the applied pressure in the throat of the grip, then the fingers and thumb will be forced into contact with the grip and, depending on the size of the hand relative to the grip, cause them to apply some torque by direct pressure or by skin torque of the web. To attempt to keep the fingers and thumb out of contact would firstly cause unnecessary muscle tension and, secondly, would eventually lead them to collapse into contact with the bow (**Fig. 3**).

Although, as with many of the situations described, the individual errors may be small in isolation, collectively they create a situation which would have a major effect. For example, the above effect, caused by using an inappropriate bow grip, combined with those discussed on pp. 112–14, would cause shooting inconsistencies, difficult to identify, as similar inconsistencies can be caused by other, more familiar, faults. The design and construction of the bow should allow the archer to use the body efficiently and effectively to shoot arrows consistently into the intended mark. If by intention, or by neglect, the bow and/or its accessories dictate by their shape or by implied instructions that any part of the human anatomy is forced to function inefficiently, then it is the equipment that must be corrected, modified or adapted to the user, not the other way round.

If the centre of dynamic limb balance does fall in the throat of the bow grip and the bow only reacts efficiently if the applied pressure is at that point, and if in attempting to achieve this the archer is forced to function unnaturally and inefficiently, the bow should be re-tillered about the centre of pressure that the archer applies most consistently and efficiently.

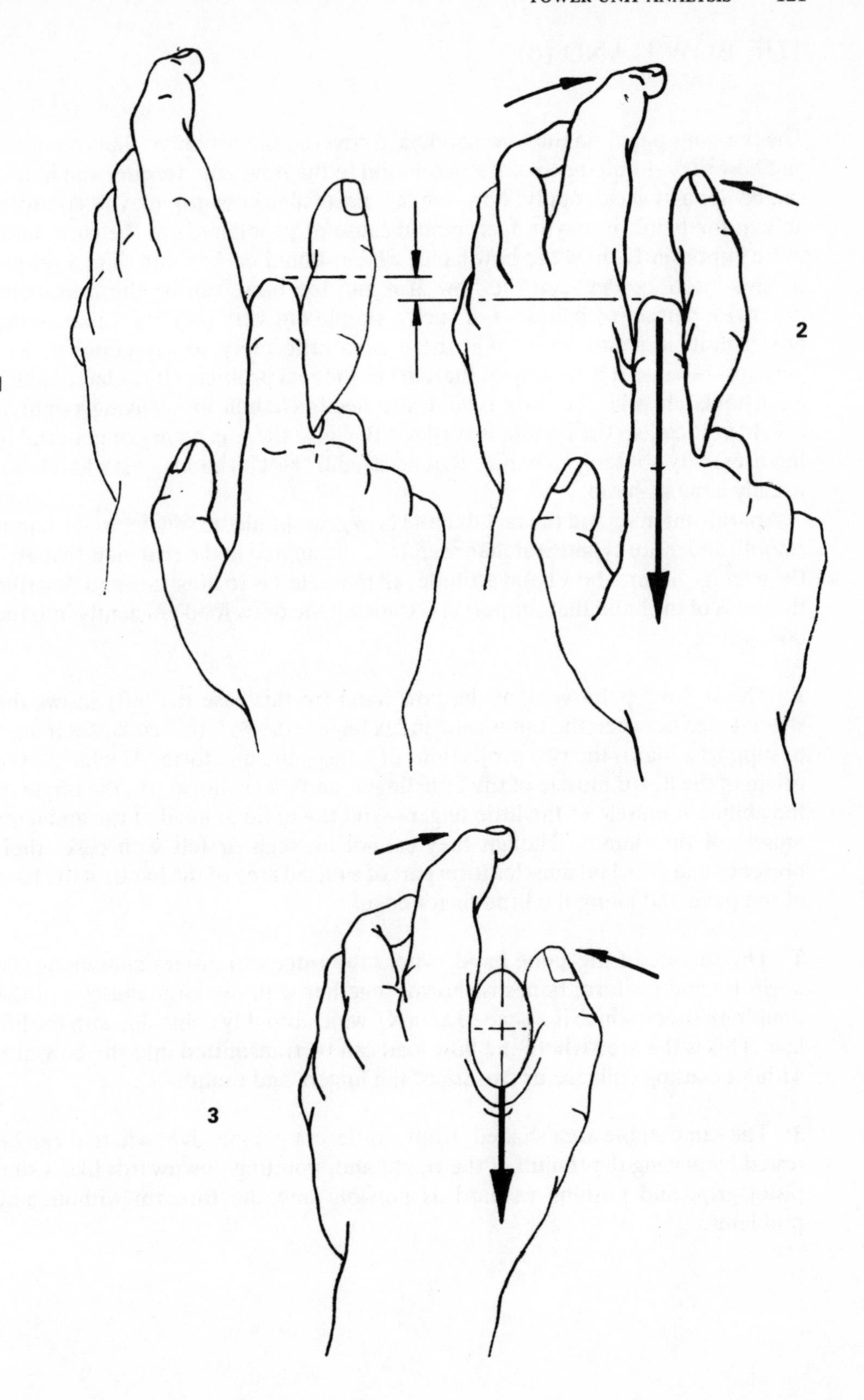
1
2
3

THE BOW HAND (6)

The previous pages on the bow hand have covered the problems that can occur and how they should be avoided in relation to the bow grip: torque, and how it can be applied accidentally; how, while a particular bow grip may fit comfortably in the hand, it may in fact, be the cause of problems, not the cure; and, more importantly, how the bow hand, which should be no more than a simple passive interface between the bow arm and the bow, can be the ruin of an otherwise perfect technique. For such a simple but very important part of the power unit, it seems a pity that there is so little more to say about it, and perhaps, because it is so simple, therein lies the real problem. It is a hand, and a hand holds a handle. The bow is held, so it needs a handle and, having a sight, it is held vertical, so the handle is vertical. Because there is plenty of material in the riser, why not sculpt a handle that fits a hand? Not all hands, just a hand, but usually a man's hand.

Apart from that, and the fact that the bow grip should be smaller in the hand, smooth and more cylindrical than sculpted, and angled in the rear view to match the average natural bow hand attitude, all that is left is to illustrate and describe the areas of the hand that support and transmit the draw load efficiently into the bow arm.

1 The skeletal palm view of the bow hand (in this case the left) shows the shaded area between the thumb and index finger (the web that collapses if used to support a load), the two projections of bone—the unciform 'A' which is the origin of the flexor muscle of the little finger, and the pisiform 'B', the origin of the abductor muscle of the little finger—and the oblique head of the abductor muscle of the thumb. Though they cannot be seen or felt with ease, their presence and attached muscles form part of a raised area of the hand, at the base of the palm and along the little finger edge.

2 The surface of the same hand, where the ridge of muscles containing the unciform and pisiform bones is shown, together with the large muscles of the thumb, between which is a shaded area 'C' which roughly coincides with the life line. This is the area where the bow load can be transmitted into the bow arm without causing collapse or closure of the fingers and thumb.

3 The same stable area shaded, from a different perspective, where it can be tested by placing the thumb of the right hand, pointing downwards like a slim pistol grip, and pushing as hard as possible into the forearm without any problems.

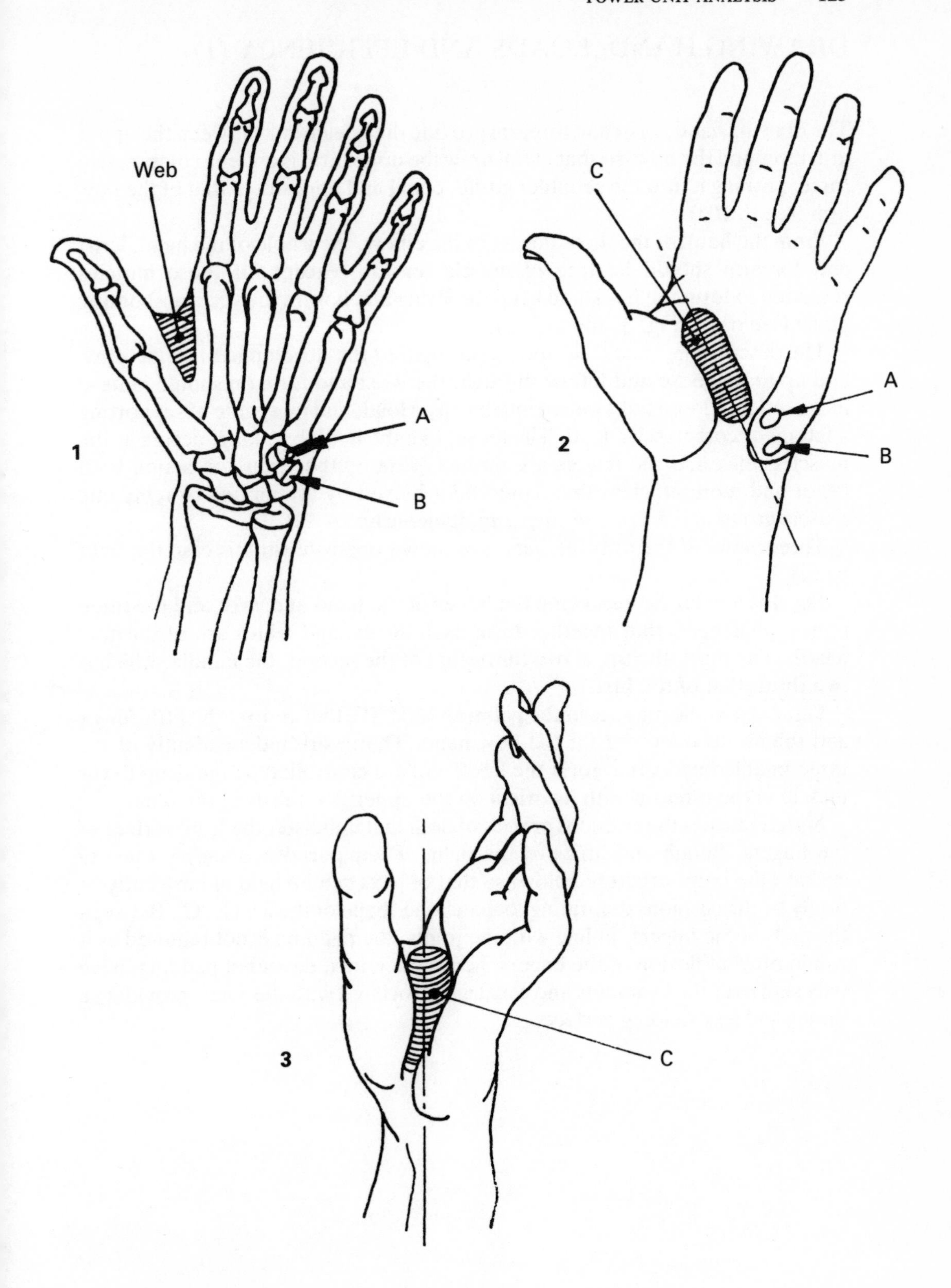
Web
A
B
1
C
A
B
2
3
C

DRAWING HAND, LOADS AND EFFICIENCY (1)

The drawing hand, wrist and forearm provide the tensile link between the upper arm lever and the bow, so that at full draw the upper arm is under a compressive force, pushing it into the shoulder girdle, equal and opposite to that of the bow arm (see p. 103).

From the hook of the three fingers to the elbow, the whole of the hand, wrist and forearm should be free of muscle tension, except for those muscles recruited to form the hook and keep the string and bow in the vertical shooting plane (see p. 55, Fig. 3, and p. 112).

The description, 'hook', is apt, as throughout the development of the draw and up to the loose and follow-through, the wrist and forearm should behave like a series of loose links pulled into line by a load, and incapable of supporting a lateral or compressive load. The loose, like the hook breaking, occurs as the muscles relax and the fingers are pushed aside by the string, an action both faster and more efficient than could be achieved by attempting to relax one muscle group and recruit another simultaneously.

Three views of the drawing hand are shown opposite (in this case the right hand).

Fig. 1 is a palm view showing the bones of the hand and wrist and the three bones, phalanges, that together form each finger, and which are of unequal length. The third, the tip, is two thirds that of the second, the middle, which is two thirds that of the first.

Fig. 2 shows the muscles in the palm, 'A' and 'B', that control the little finger and thumb, as discussed for the bow hand. They work independently of the three middle fingers that form the hook and are controlled by the deep flexor muscle in the forearm with its origin on the upper two thirds of the ulna.

Fig. 3 indicates the cushions or pads of flesh that upholster the front surface of the fingers, thumb and areas of the palm. Their purpose is simply that: to cushion the bony structure below, so that objects can be held either gently or firmly by the cushions deforming to match the shape of the article 'C'. Between the pads of the fingers, in line with the joints, the padding is not required as it would prevent flexion of the fingers; hence the joints, devoid of padding, have only skin over the ligaments and cartilage associated with the joint, providing a firmer and less yielding surface.

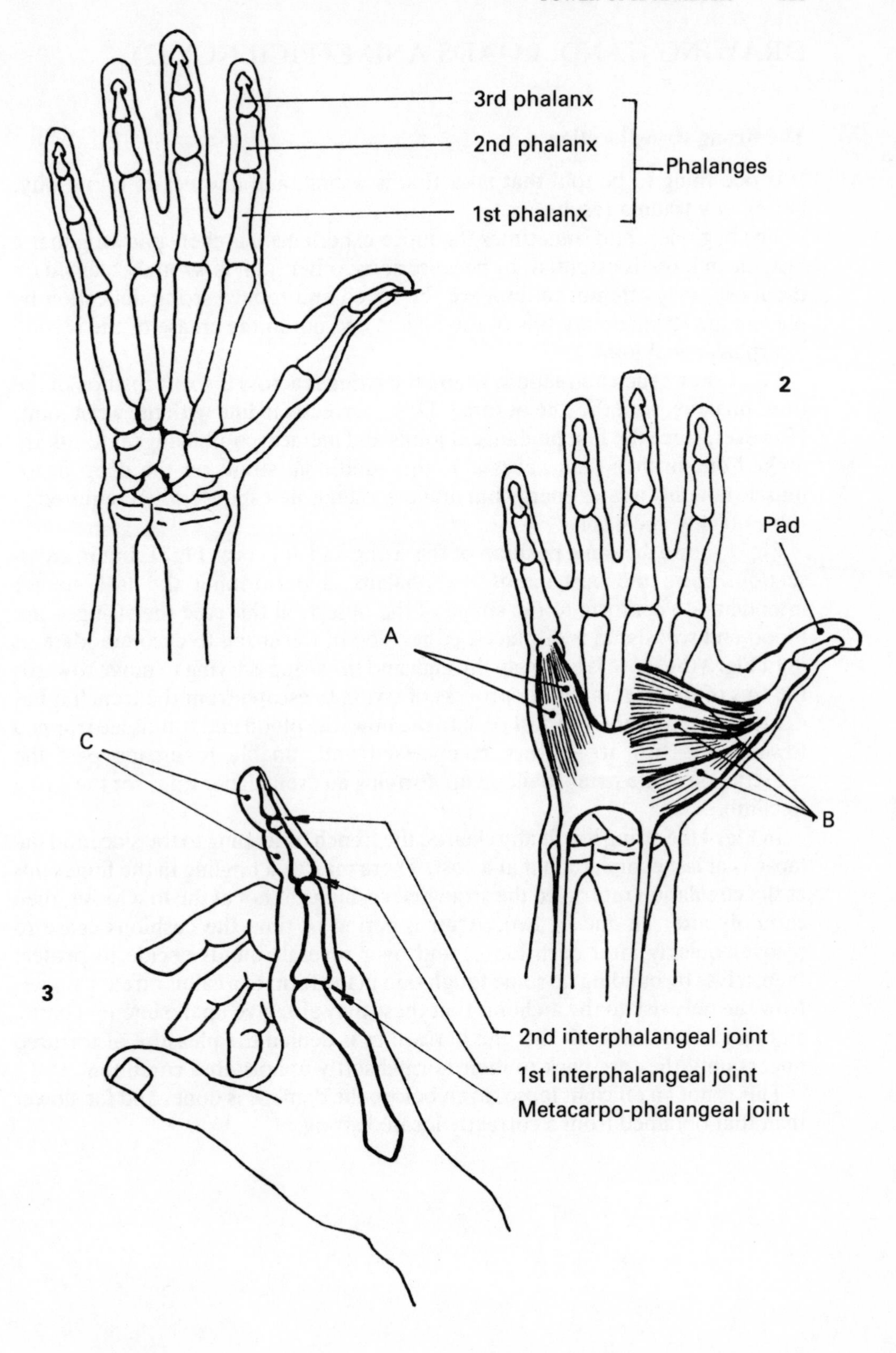
3rd phalanx
2nd phalanx
Phalanges
1st phalanx
1
2
Pad
A
B
C
3
2nd interphalangeal joint
1st interphalangeal joint
Metacarpo-phalangeal joint

DRAWING HAND, LOADS AND EFFICIENCY (2)

The wrong string location

It is one thing to be told that an action is wrong, and another to know why, before any trauma results.

The beginner, and sometimes the more experienced archer, knowing that a fast, clean loose is essential, or because some other fault is wrongly blamed on the loose, may attempt to improve the speed and reduce string deflection by placing the string on the tips of the fingers and not in the crease of the second interphalangeal joint.

Fig. 1 shows such a situation, where the string is across the soft cushion of the third phalanx, with the line of force, DFL, correctly in line with the wrist joint. However, since the first phalangeal joints and metacarpo-phalangeal joints are arched out further than necessary, the additional strain on the deep flexor muscle not only wastes energy but induces a sluggish response when required to relax quickly and easily.

Fig. 2 shows the same position of the string and fingers as **Fig. 1**, but in cross-section. Here the cushion of the phalanx is performing the task nature intended—to conform to the shape of the object, in this case the string—and blood and soft tissue is displaced either side of the string to accommodate it.

In **Fig. 3** the loose is half-way through and the string is trying to move towards the tips of the fingers. In the process of trying to escape from the trench it has made for itself by the shortest path to the bow, the blood and soft tissue trapped towards the tips are further compressed and, unable to escape past the constriction of the string, balloon up, forming an even higher ridge for the string to climb.

In **Fig. 4** the string has finally cleared the trench by leaping to the side, and the loose is at last complete, but at a cost. There may be a tingling in the finger tips as the circulation returns to the strangled cushions, if not at the first loose, then certainly after an end or two. After a period of time the cushions cease to recover quickly after each loose, and over several rounds decide to protect themselves by building up some tough skin in the form of a callus on each finger. Now the only risk to the archer is that these may also give up the unequal battle and tear, with the result that the performer is denied the pleasure of tortured fingers until they are back to their normal softly upholstered condition.

This is not an efficient loose, even before the damage is done, and far slower than that obtained from a correctly located string.

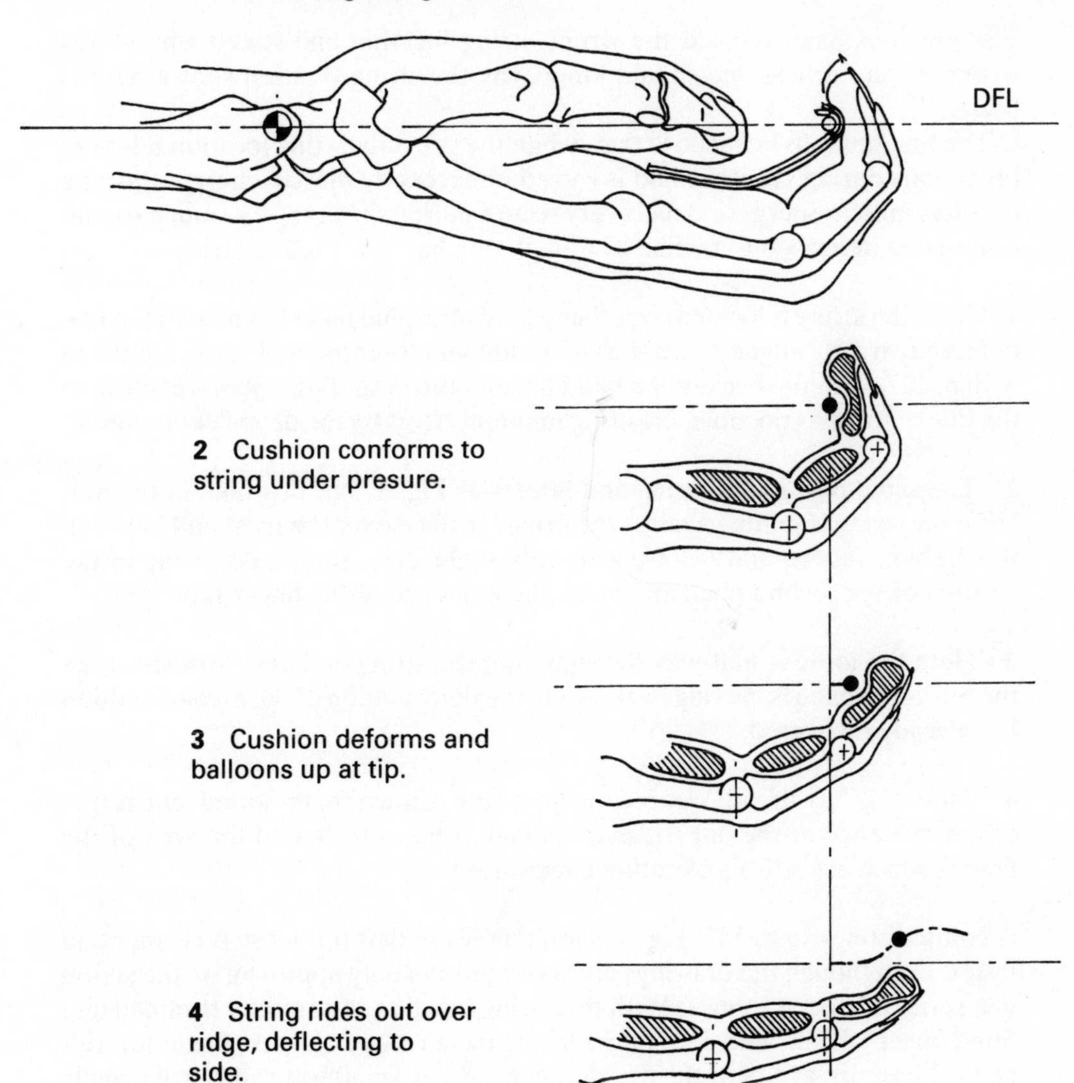

1 The wrong string location.

2 Cushion conforms to string under presure.

3 Cushion deforms and balloons up at tip.

4 String rides out over ridge, deflecting to side.

DRAWING HAND, LOADS AND EFFICIENCY (3)

The correct string location

The previous page showed the wrong string location and stated why it was wrong, so in fairness one should know why the string location shown here is better.

The first point to be made is that, while the previous string location felt very precarious during the draw and involved unnecessary muscle energy, this one uses less muscle energy and feels very secure during the draw—so much so that it has been described as feeling as though one has 'a fist full of string'.

1 Here the string is located over the second interphalangeal joint with the line of force correctly aligned with the wrist joint and forearm, and, by comparison with p. 127, with the back of the hand flat and the other finger joints as close to the line of force as possible, ensuring minimal effort by the deep flexor muscle.

2 The same position of string and fingers as **Fig. 1**, but this time in section. Here the string is pulling against the firmer surface over the joint and between the cushions above and below, with only slight deformation occurring in the cushion of the second phalanx, under the influence of the finger tab.

3 Here the loose is half-way through, and the string is sliding forwards over the tab as the hand is moving back, while the deformation of the second cushion has already recovered.

4 The string has already cleared the finger tab, shown chain-dotted, and is free of the influence of the fingers, even though it has not cleared the area of the fingers which are still accelerating backwards.

A comparison with p. 127, Fig. 4, should indicate that this loose is cleaner and faster, even though the drawings are static and can only approximate the action in a series of frozen frames. With this string location, a correctly trimmed and fitted finger tab and with each finger taking its fair share of work, finger injuries and calluses are avoided; the development of any small soft callus will usually indicate an ill-fitting tab or a finger not taking its fair share of work and being rubbed by the passing string instead of being flung free by it. In general, a callus is the result of friction, not load, hence the reason for the calluses on the previous page. The string did not fling the fingers away so much as drag over them.

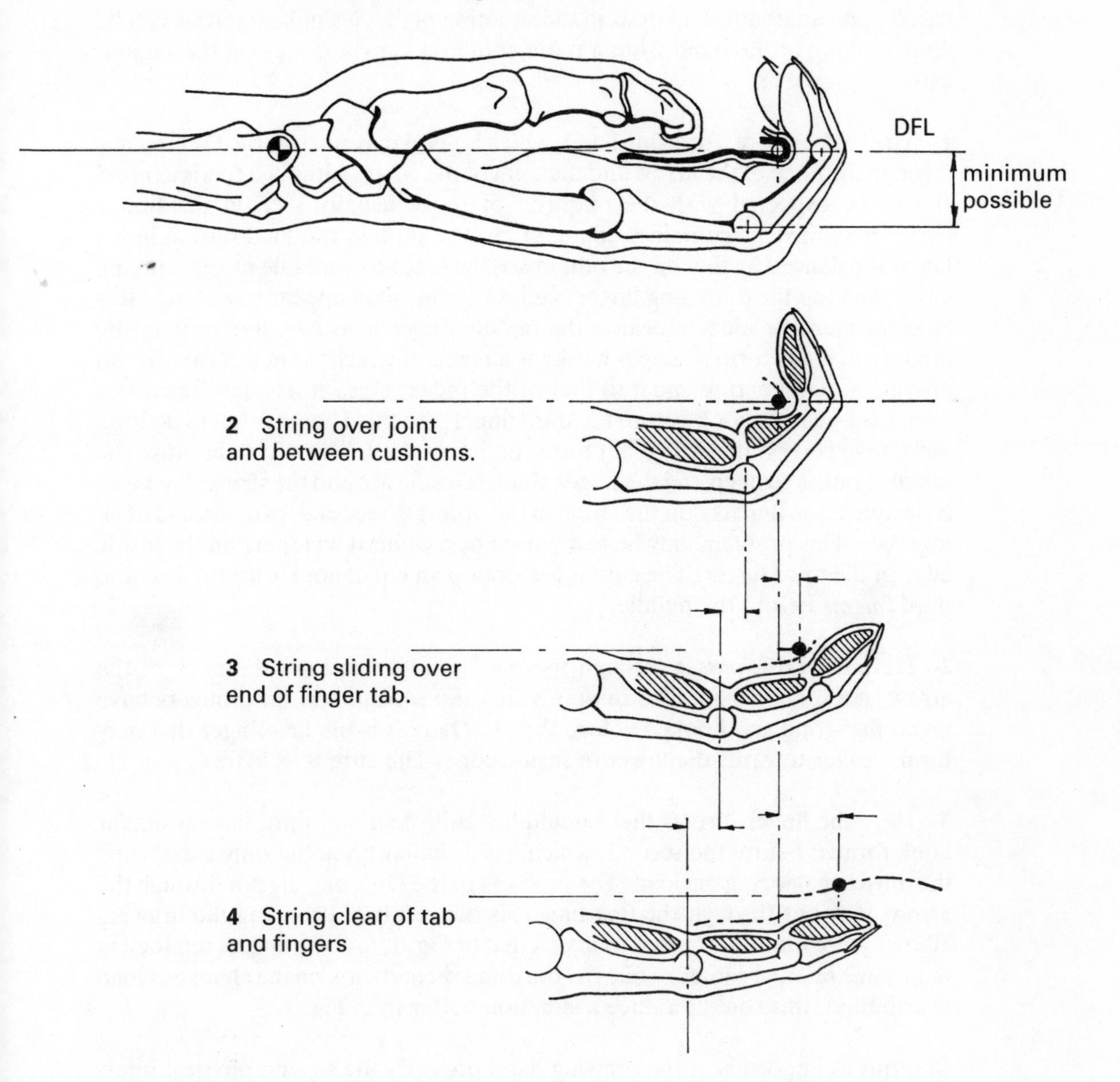
1 The correction string location.
DFL
minimum
possible
2 String over joint
and between cushions.
3 String sliding over
end of finger tab.
4 String clear of tab
and fingers

DRAWING HAND, LOADS AND EFFICIENCY (4)

Having had a look at the drawing hand from above and considered some faults based upon anatomical analysis in the shooting plane, a similar exercise can be done looking at the hand from a more common viewpoint, along the sagittal axis.

1 The back view of a drawing hand, which is good inasmuch as the DFL passes through the nock of the arrow and the joint of the wrist. Although this is as good as can be expected with the majority of those usually seen in the better performers, it does contain a common fault: although the load on the index finger is balanced by that on the other two, the second or middle finger is taking more than the third, or ring finger, and while this may appear trivial, it is less efficient than the ideal. Because the middle finger is usually longer than the other two, it can form a deeper hook, as a result of which, as in this case, it can provide a load-bearing equal to that of the index; since it has developed this deep load-bearing hook before the third finger, the third finger is left to do little more than rest on the string and forms no hook at all. Therefore, because the middle hook is so deep and the finger almost closing around the string, the loose is slowed as the fingers quit the string in the order, three, one, two, instead of all together. This problem may be recognised by a callus developing on the inside edge of the third finger. The cure is to develop an equal hook with the first and third fingers before the middle.

2 Here the DFL passes through the middle finger and not the nock of the arrow, not a good sign. The reason is that the second and third fingers have taken the string and hooked before the first; here it is the first finger that may form a callus towards the lower or inside edge. The cure is as before.

3 Here the fingers are as they should be. Both first and third have a similar hook formed before the second, which has a similar hook but only supporting the third in balancing the load. The problem of the DFL passing not through the arrow nock but through the first finger, is the result of dropping the drawing elbow. Were the elbow raised to match that of **Fig. 1**, and the fingers retained in their same relative contact while the third and second took on the change in load distribution, this could produce a situation better than **Fig. 1**.

In terms of importance, the drawing hand provides the second physical interface with the bow, the first being the bow hand. The drawing hand only ranks a very close second, simply because it leaves the bow string while the bow hand is still able to ruin an otherwise perfect loose.

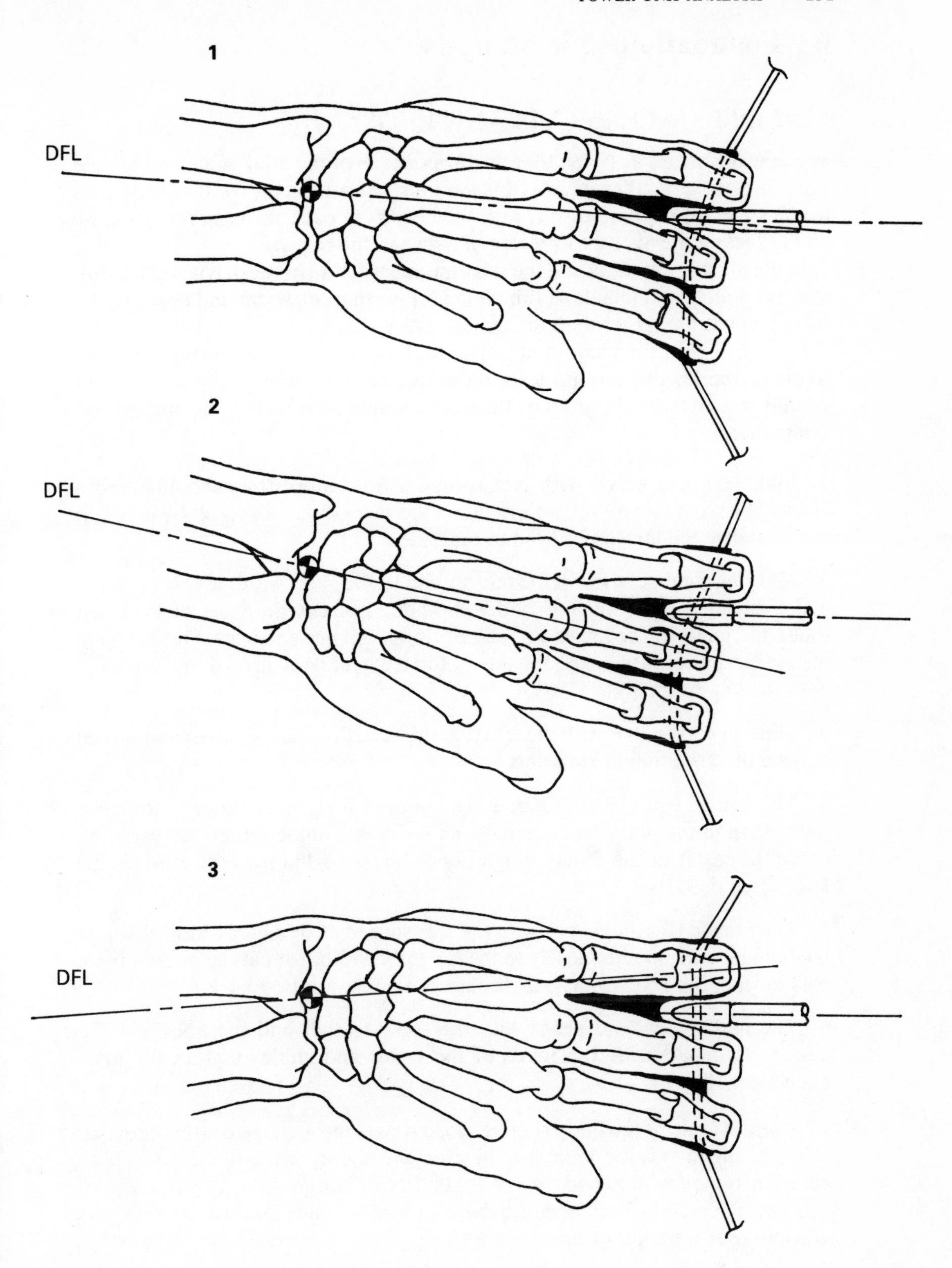
1
DFL
2
DFL
3
DFL

6 Foundation Unit Analysis

MALE/FEMALE PELVIS AND LEGS

We saw in Chapter 1, p. 39, that the proportions of the adult male and female skeletons are very different, and this was illustrated using the width of the pelvis as the standard of comparison, with the heights of each skeleton representing and reflecting the average differential between the sexes.

In the illustrations opposite the skeletal construction of the pelvis and legs are those of a male and female of similar height, so that the width and depth of the female pelvis are larger than the male.

In each Figure the chain-dotted lines extending vertically through the ball joints of the hips to ground level represent the direction of the bodyweight equally shared and supported by the legs, assuming the body to be upright and symmetrical.

1 Male legs and pelvis with feet spread a little more than shoulder-width apart. The second overlaid outline shows the swing-boat action of the pelvis, if in this stance the hips are moved to one side.

2 Male legs and pelvis with the feet spread to shoulder width which, with the male, having proportionately wider shoulders, places the lines of load just inside the joints of the knees and ankles. If, as will be seen later, the feet were placed hip-joint width apart, the line of force would pass through the centre of both the knee and ankle joints.

3 Male legs and pelvis with the feet together and the lines of force passing well outside the knee and ankle joints.

4 The female equivalent of **Fig. 1**. The lines of force pass closer to the knee joints than in the male version, and well inside the ankle joints, the variation being the result of the female thigh bones being angled inwards towards the knees (see p. 39).

5 The female legs and pelvis with the feet spaced at shoulder width which, in the female, corresponds closely to the hip joint width, so that the lines of force pass outside the knee joints but through the ankle joints.

6 The female legs and pelvis with the feet together and the lines of force passing farther outside the joints of the knees and ankles than in the male equivalent (**Fig. 3**).

As a general rule, if the line of applied load passes through the centre of several joints in alignment, the joints will be efficient as they will only be exposed to compressive loads. When the line of applied load diverges from a joint, the joint will be subjected to both compressive and torque loads and will become less efficient over a period of time.

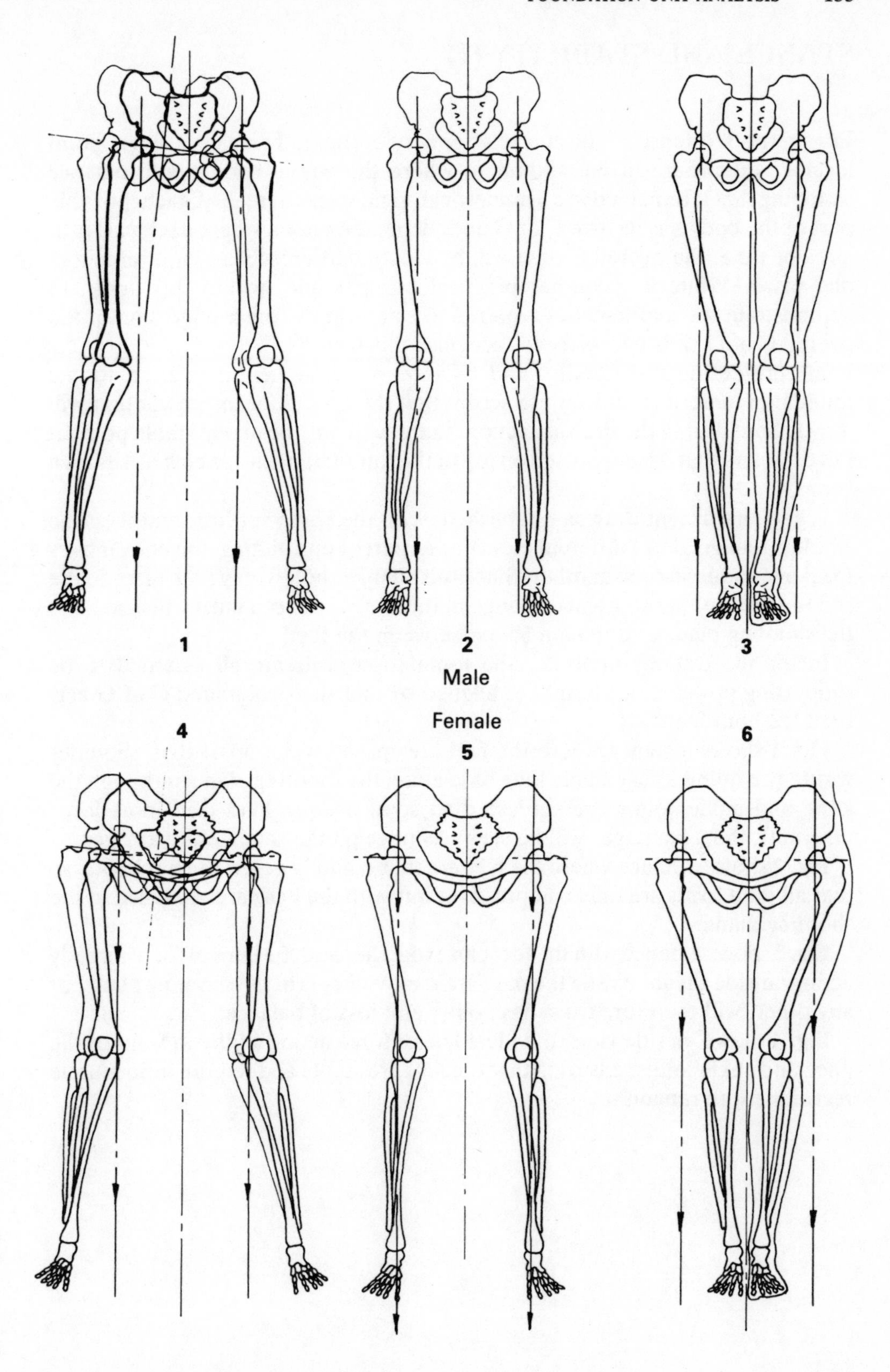
1
2
3
Male
Female
4
5
6

STANCE AND STABILITY (1)

In general, reference to the centre of gravity of the body means a single point located somewhere in the abdomen, where the whole body would balance assuming that it remained in a symmetrical, rigid state. In reality, each movable part of the body has its own C of G and, depending upon where each part is at any one time, the overall C of G will be located differently and not remain in one place. While it is neither practical nor possible, within this book, to demonstrate the mathematics required to establish the precise location of the overall C of G, it is necessary to recognise this fact.

In considering the stability and balance of an archer in relation to the foundation unit, it is sufficient to accept that the C of G for the power unit will move about during the drawing action, that it will only be at one stable point at full draw and that it is supported on top of the foundation unit, which has its own C of G.

When an efficient draw is established, with the spine vertical, and then the whole is realigned to a different elevation as part of unit aiming, the body moves from one stable state to another. Since this change should only take place in the shooting plane, the combined change in the C of G of both units will also be in the shooting plane and remain acting between the feet.

In the illustrations opposite, the foundation units are all assumed to be supporting power unit assemblies aligned so that their combined C of G acts between both feet.

Fig. 1 shows a stance where the feet are spaced wider apart than shoulder width, providing a very stable long base along the shooting plane; although the knee and ankle joints are subjected to some torque load (see inset force diagram), the advantages will be seen to outweigh the small disadvantages.

Fig. 2 shows a stance where the feet are immediately below the hip joints, so that all joint loads are only compressive, but with the base area reduced in the shooting plane.

Fig. 3 shows a stance with the feet close together and the lines of force already acting outside the joints and the base area; movements in the shooting plane, or any other, will therefore cause instability and loss of balance.

Fig. 4 shows, in side view, the ideal line of force acting a little in front of the knee and ankle joints, ensuring that the legs are stable and require little muscle recruitment to remain so.

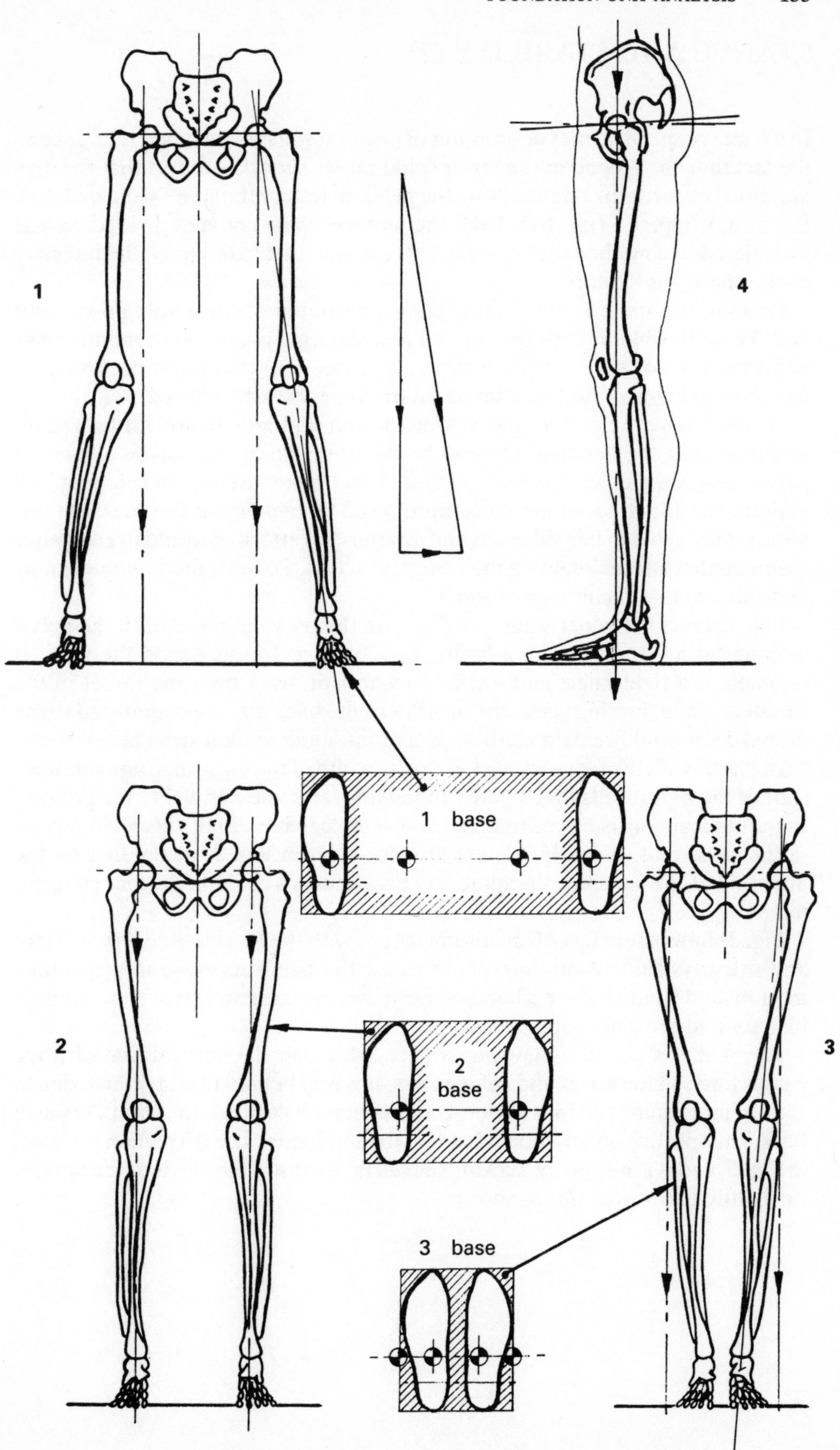
1
4
1 base
2
2
base
3
3 base

STANCE AND STABILITY (2)

In Chapter 4, p. 68, a brief description of postural collapse included reference to the fact that an 'S' bend of the lower spine causes such discomfort that the hips are thrust towards the target, tilting the pelvis to reduce the spine's angle of exit. Later, in Chapter 5 (pp. 102–104), the uniform spine and muscle loading was considered and methods of achieving a technique that maintained the integrity of the spine was explored.

Because the spine is the main supporting column of the whole power unit and, being flexible in both the sagittal and shooting planes, is prone to abuse and the cause of severe back trouble, it is essential that all unnecessary or unbalanced loads should be eliminated or, at very least, reduced.

As mentioned on p. 106, the instructions on unit aiming are a little vague, saying merely, 'by bending sideways at the waist'. Since the waist is above the pelvis, any muscles of the back recruited and committed to developing and maintaining the draw would be compromised by bending at the waist, as this requires the spine to flex sideways and any muscles attached would need to alter their length while maintaining their original action. Possibly this is why so many find this action difficult to perform.

Fig. 1 shows the wider stance of Fig. 1 on the previous page, with the pelvis moving from side to side in a 'swing boat' action. In this action the spine is retained at a right angle and inclines towards or away from the target in the shooting plane, in which case any muscles of the back that are committed to the draw action would remain unaffected and the spine remain straight.

In **Fig. 2**, with the feet spaced close to the width of the hip joints, any sideways shift of the hips results in the pelvis remaining level and parallel to the ground, so that unit aiming is forced to occur above the pelvis, with the associated bend in the spine and so on. If the feet are closer, as in **Fig. 3**, depending on the direction of the hip shift, the spine and back muscles could be further compromised.

Fig. 3 shows the effect of an upright stance with the feet close together. Here any sideways shift of the hips could cause the pelvis to move in a 'pitching motion' and would induce a bend in the spine, as the archer strove to maintain balance and prevent toppling over.

Fig. 4 shows the side elevation where, although the vertical line of force passes through the knees and ankle joints, it is well behind the hip joints, due to the archer pushing the hips forwards to maintain balance as the shoulders lean back, thus putting an additional load on the hip joints. The correction is shown in **Fig. 5**, and is achieved by 'tucking the tail in' to return the pelvis to the upright or slightly backwards tilt, as shown.

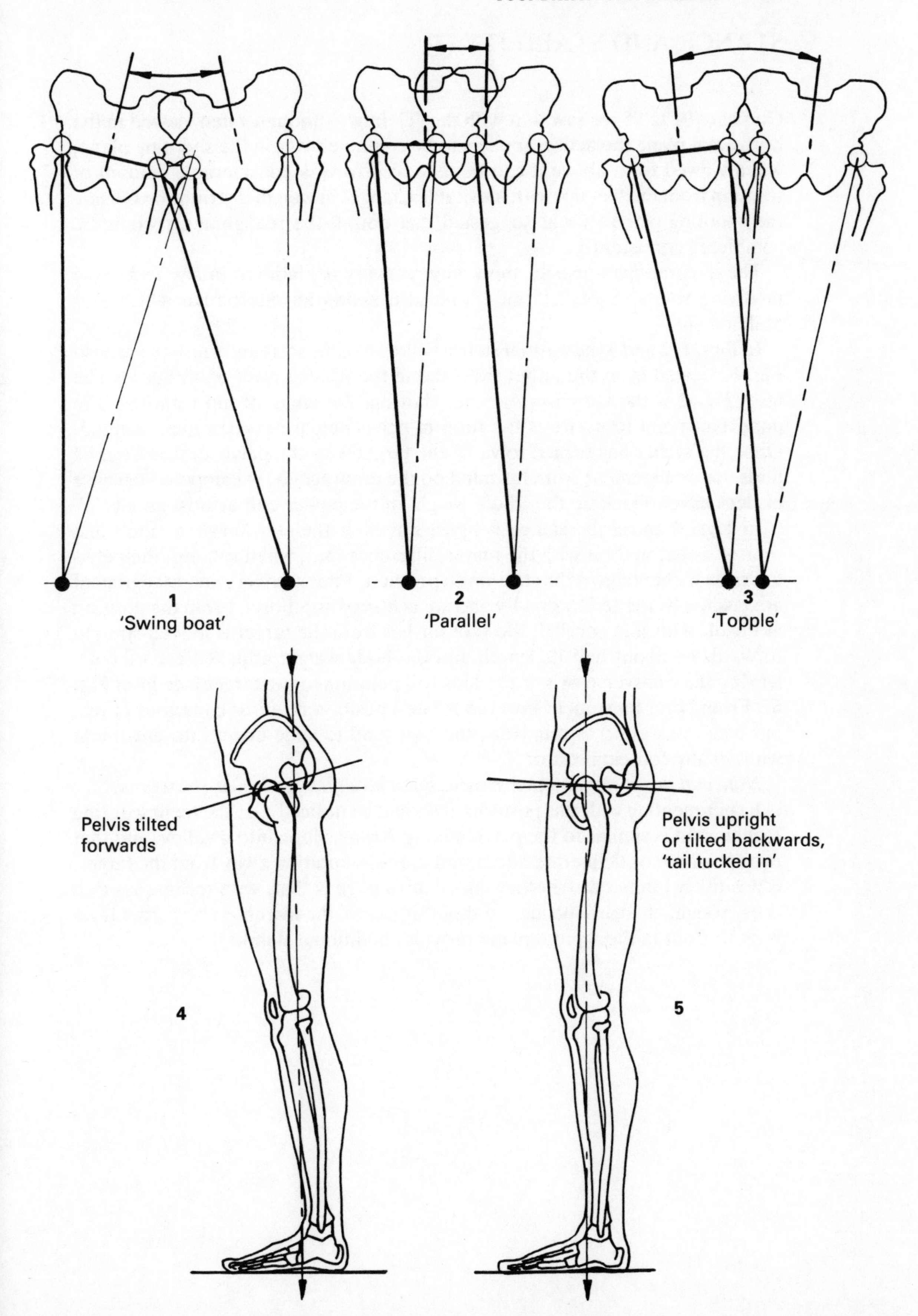
1
'Swing boat'
2
'Parallel'
3
'Topple'
Pelvis tilted
forwards
Pelvis upright
or tilted backwards,
'tail tucked in'
4
5

STANCE AND STABILITY (3)

On pages 92 to 95 we saw that with the 'T' draw, although when viewed in the horizontal plane the action appears to be contained within the shooting plane, when viewed from above it can be seen to involve a considerable amount of rotation from the feet up, with inevitable changes in weight distribution outside the shooting plane. It was suggested that not all the realignments would be completed consistently.

The illustrations opposite show why recovery is hindered in any technique involving rotations of the body, and also shows an alternative which aids realignment.

In **Figs. 1**, **2** and **3** the normal stance is shown in the start and finish position in **Fig. 1**, viewed from the target side, and in the rotated position in **Fig. 3**. The inset **Fig. 2** is the view from above, showing the angle of hip rotation. The important point to notice is the drop in pelvis height between **Figs. 1** and **3**. Once the archer has turned towards the target with the pelvis descending, he finds that realignment, with his mind on the draw action, is hampered because his legs have to jack up the whole weight of the power unit against gravity.

In **Figs. 4** and **5** the stance is again shown at the start/finish position and rotated as before, but with the major difference that, when rotated, the pelvis has risen higher than at the start/finish position. Thus recovery and realignment are positively assisted by gravity and are achieved as follows. From the position at **Fig. 1**, with feet parallel, the foot farther from the target is moved straight forwards by about half its length and the body weight adjusted accordingly, leaving the transverse axis of the hips still pointing to the target (see inset **Fig. 6**). From here, movement into the rotated position requires conscious effort, but when this effort is removed, the hips tend to slide down into alignment without any conscious effort.

Note that this is not an open stance, but a modified square or rhomboid.

Experimenting with this position, it should be noticed that the feeling during realignment is similar to the pelvis sliding down a slope into a valley, and that over-rotation, or deliberate attempted opposite rotation away from the target, is positively inhibited. Another added advantage is that, with techniques that cause weight changes outside the shooting plane, the increased base area from back to front in the sagittal plane provides additional stability.

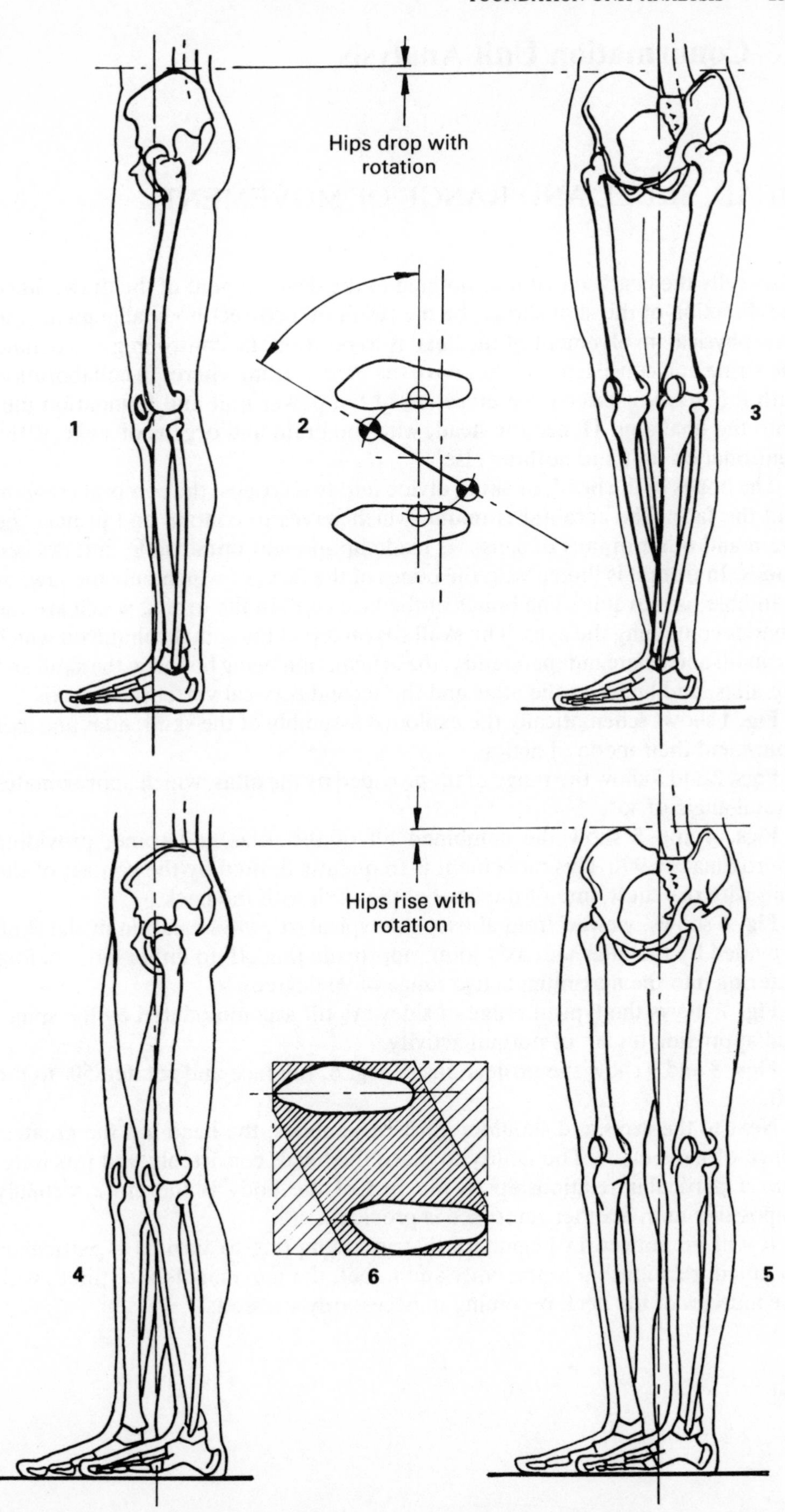
Hips drop with
rotation
1
2
3
Hips rise with
rotation
4
6
5

7 Confirmation Unit Analysis

HEAD, SKULL AND RANGE OF MOVEMENT

Physically the head contributes nothing to the development of the draw. Since the direction of the shot should be the result of a correct body alignment, the only physical involvement of the head is to position the controlling eye behind the string at a consistent height above the arrow, from where, in collaboration with the brain, it directs the elevation of the power unit and foundation unit onto the final aim. Hence the head, with the brain and organs of sight, is the confirmation unit and nothing else.

The bones of the head, or skull, divide into two groups, the cerebral cranium and the face. The cerebral cranium, which serves to contain and protect the brain and other organs of sense, is made up of eight immovable, interlocked bones. In front it is linked with the bones of the face, of which only the jaw, or mandible, is movable. The bones of the face contain the orbits, which are the cavities containing the eyes. The skull sits on top of the spinal column on which it can tilt and rotate independently, the articulation being between the skull and the atlas, and between the atlas and the second cervical vertebra, the axis.

Fig. 1 shows schematically the exploded assembly of the skull, atlas and axis bones and their mode of action.

Figs. 2 and **3** show the range of tilt provided by the atlas, which approximates a total angle of 45°.

Figs. 4 and **5** show the combined tilt of the atlas and spine, providing approximately 90°. This movement is frequently limited by the contact of the chin with the chest, and of the base of the skull with the neck.

Fig. 6 shows, viewed from above, the typical sideways rotation of the skull provided by the atlas and axis joint, approximating 50° to either side, before entering into the maximum active range of 90 degrees.

Fig. 7 shows the typical range of sideways tilt accommodated by the spine, and approximates 30° of normal activity.

Figs. 8 and **9** show the projections of **Fig. 6**, full face and rotated 50° to the left.

Next to the arms and shoulder girdle assemblies, the head has the greatest range of movement. The ability to place the head, consistenly and precisely, into a particular relationship to the rest of the body is therefore virtually impossible until another reference is provided.

It will be noticed in beginners that in attempting to turn to a particular, assumed, relationship to the body and target, the movements are stilted, with the muscles of the neck becoming unnecessarily stressed.

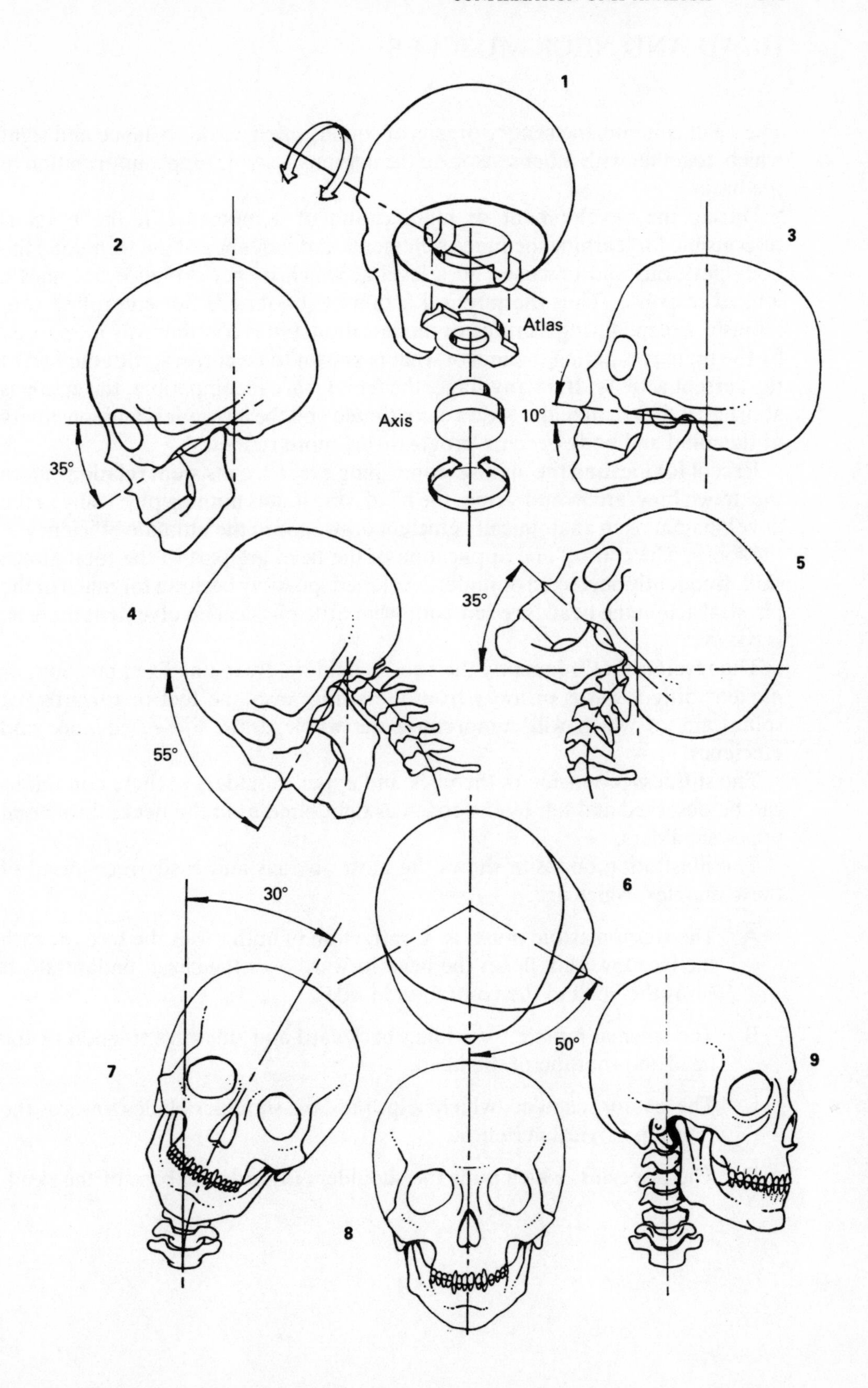
1
2
3
Atlas
Axis
10°
35°
4
5
35°
55°
6
30°
50°
7
8
9

HEAD AND NECK MUSCLES

The head contains the senory organs of sound, smell, taste, balance and sight which, together with other sensors of the nervous system, supply information to the brain.

During the development or modification of a motor skill, the brain is responsible for learning the precise elements and sequence of the technique the body performs and practises, to a level at which its performance becomes a unified response. Thus the physical action of shooting is not controlled consciously, except during learning or modification, but is continuously monitored by the brain comparing the feel of what is known to be correct, with the feel of the current activity. If, at any stage, the feelings are incompatible, the action is aborted; if they match, the action is continued and the awareness and sensitivity of the mind and body become progressively more refined.

Except for locating the aiming, controlling eye in a consistent relationship to the drawn bow, arrow and string, the head contributes nothing physically to the development of an anatomically efficient draw, nor to the ultimate efficiency of the loose. The control and application of the head are part of the total motor skill, frequently neglected or underdeveloped, possibly because for much of the physical action the head is redundant; what little physical involvement there is, is passive.

The result is that frequently the head is held rigidly in one fixed position, or moved stiffly towards or away from the string, over the feet or towards the spine, any of which will compromise the whole draw, loose sequence and efficiency.

The stiffness or tension in the neck and upper shoulders in these conditions can be observed and felt by the coach as tight bundles in the neck, throat and upper shoulders.

The illustration opposite shows the most obvious and easily recognised of these muscles, which are:

A The sternomastoid muscles. Contraction of both raises the face or, with the face lowered, flexes the head forward over the chest; unilaterally it turns the head to the contralateral side.

B The splenial muscle, providing backward and sideways traction of the head and rotation of the head.

C The levator scapulae, which helps raise the shoulder blades towards the four top cervical vertebrae.

D The trapezius, which pulls the shoulders towards the base of the skull.

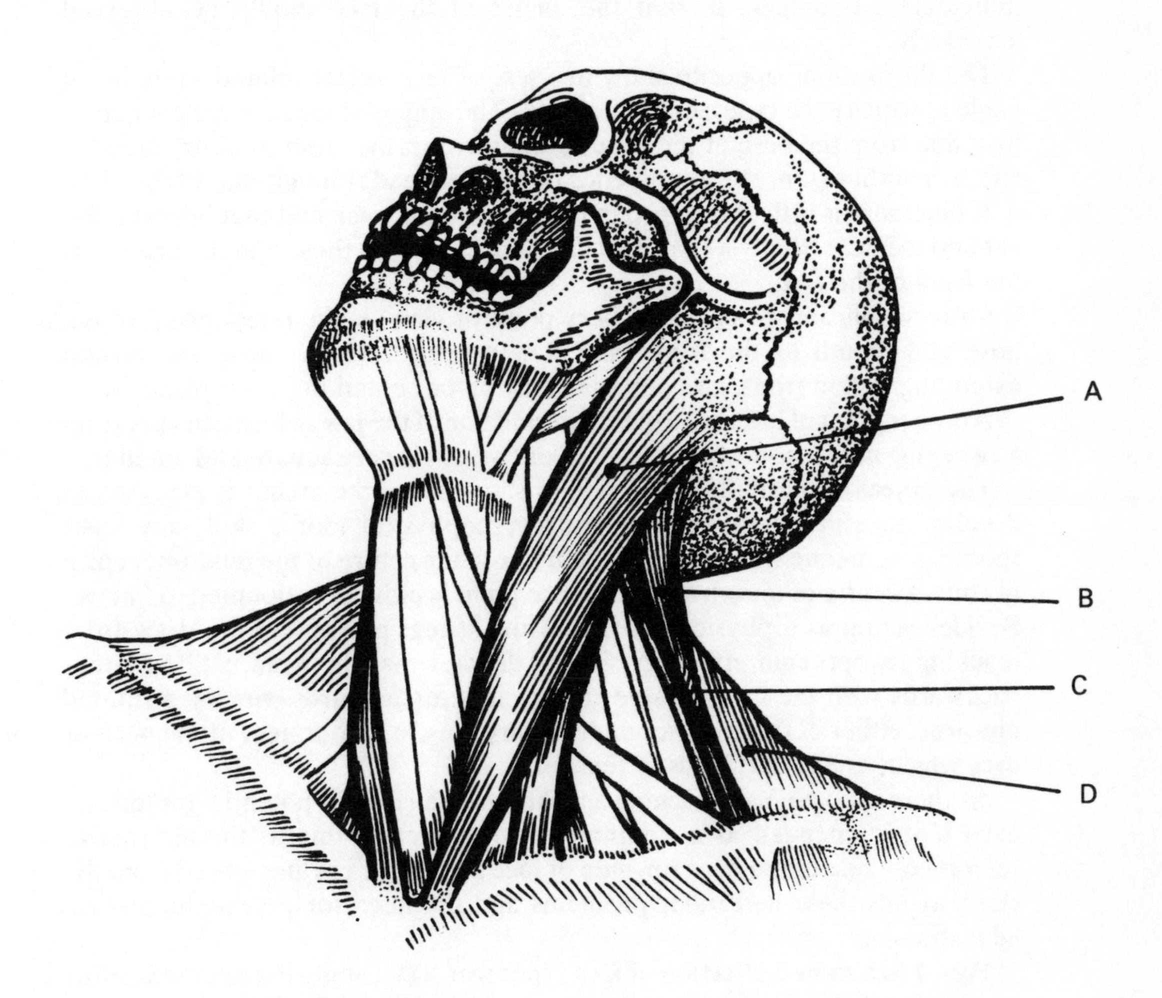

Obvious areas where stress or tension can be detected.

HEAD, NECK AND FACE ANGLES

The face angles depend on the type to which a person belongs. There are also individual differences, so that the angles of the face should be observed accurately.

The illustrations opposite show five sets of face angles related to the neck angle at which each type carries the head. The angles of the face are compared by a line from the base of the nose spine, through the outer auditory meatus, and by another from the prominence of the forehead through that of the chin.

While there is little difference in the angle of the neck and that between the ear and the nose, there is a marked difference between those and the line down the front of the face.

More significant, from the archery point of view, is the relationship of the nose and mouth to the front face plane: some have the nose and mouth extending well in front, and others mainly on or behind the front plane.

Another point of interest is the shape and line of the jaw, which can vary from a sweeping curve from chin to ear, to one which is very square and angular.

The object of these illustrations is to show that if the archer is expected to develop an efficient anatomical and psychophysical motor skill, any basic shooting technique which requires him to use the centre of the nose tip, centre of chin or centre of mouth as a reference point is ultimately doomed to failure. Besides acting as a physical barrier to the string, preventing the draw from reaching its optimum efficiency, it also dictates that the head is tilted either backwards with the eyes rotated downwards, or forwards with eyes rotated upwards; either of these causes unnecessary muscle recruitment of the neck or eyes which, as a result, leads to tension.

As there is no point in teaching a technique which has a potential for failure, even if it is intended as a stepping stone to greater things, the alternative reference—side of the nose tip, side of face and under jawline—used from the start, avoids these and other problems and the need for psychophysical re-education later on.

Figs. 1 to **5** show a selection of face types which can apply to either sex, while **Figs. 6** and **7** show two of the above types, **Figs. 2** and **5**, using a centre face alignment and under chin reference. In **Fig. 6** the neck is forced back and the eyes rotated down, while **Fig. 7** has the neck strained forwards with the eyes rolled upwards. (See also Figs. 6 and 7, p. 149.

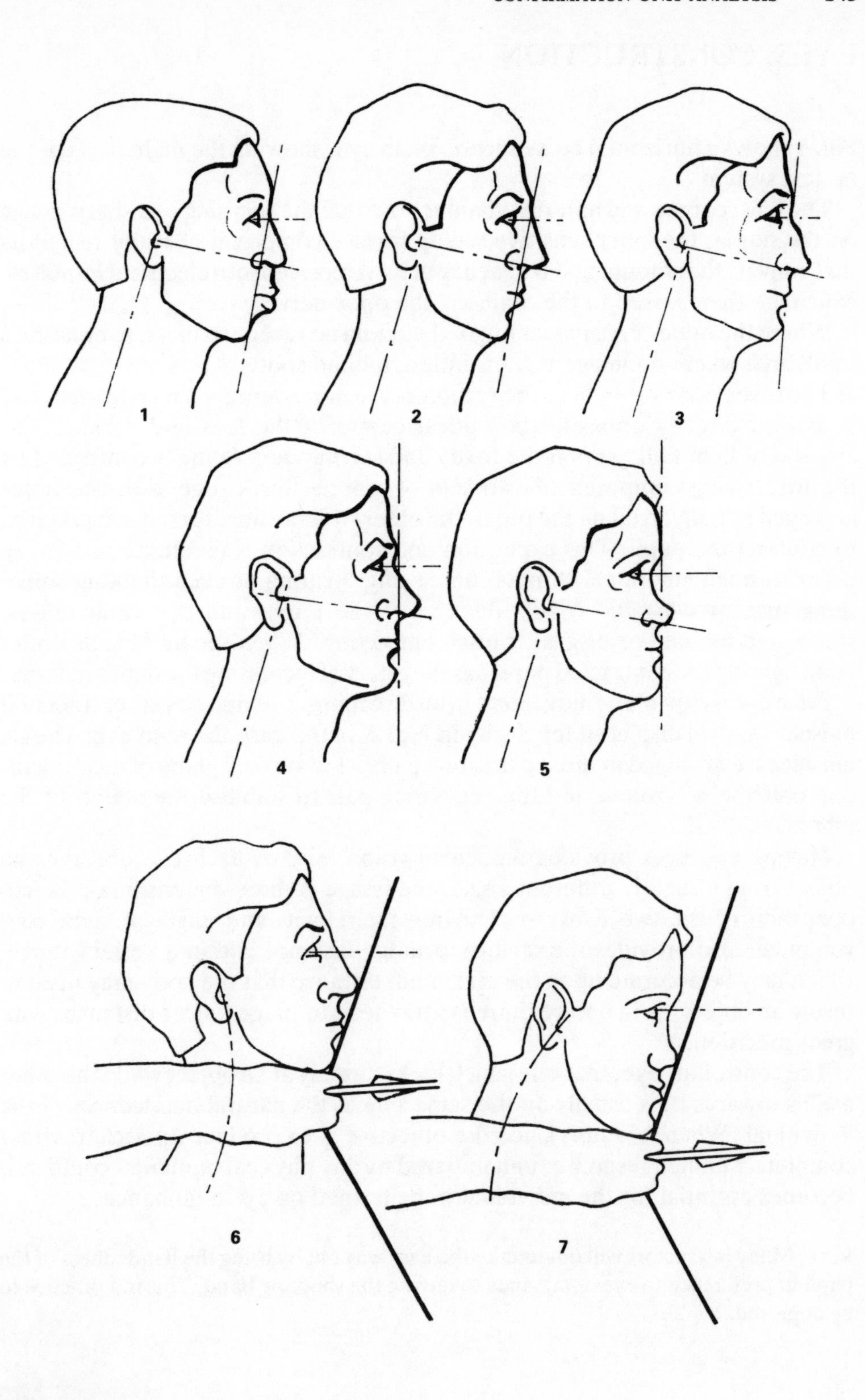
1
2
3
4
5
6
7

EYES, CONSTRUCTION

Fig. 1 shows a horizontal cross-section of an eye, showing the main parts of the optical system.

The lens, cornea and anterior chamber provide the focusing of a sharp image on the retina, the inner sensitive seeing surface composed of many receptors that convert the amount and frequency of light received into electrical impulses, which are then passed to the brain via the optic nerve.

Where the optic nerve passes out of the retina no receptors exist, so creating a small area where no image is transmitted, a blind spot.

The fovea is an area where the receptors are more densely concentrated, and is located directly opposite the optical centre of the lens and cornea. The amount of light falling upon the fovea and surrounding retina is controlled by the iris, a ring composed of two sets of muscle fibres, one with the fibres arranged radially to dilate the pupil, the other with the fibres arrange circularly, to contract the pupil. This expansion and contraction is involuntary, but can occur through emotional stimulation: seeing, hearing or even thinking something nice or desirable causes dilation of the pupil, and the same senses, stimulated by hate or disgust, cause contraction. When seeing objects under good lighting the contracted pupil has the effect of increasing the depth of focus.

Each eye is capable of movement in all directions, provided by six extraocular muscles, shown displaced for clarity in **Fig. 2**, in this case the right eye. The six muscles are arranged in three pairs, one pair in the vertical plane of movement, one pair the horizontal and the remaining pair to stabilise the action of the others.

Having two eyes provides binocular vision, and as each eye observes an object from a slightly different angle, the image is three-dimensional; the co-operation of the two eyes, in changing their focus and angle of sight convergence, also provides the facility to judge distance within a certain range, which may be accurate up to the maximum distance that the body may need to throw an object, as in nature there is little need to judge longer distances with great precision.

The controlling eye, that one which looks directly at an object while the other angles towards it, is usually on the same side as the natural handedness of the individual. When it is not, since the objective is to produce an archer with a completely unified response, unhampered by any physical or mental conflict, it becomes essential for the individual to be trained on eye dominance.

NOTE: Many instructors will opt to take the easy way out by using the handedness of the pupil in preference to eye dominance to dictate the shooting hand. This is a practice to be deplored.

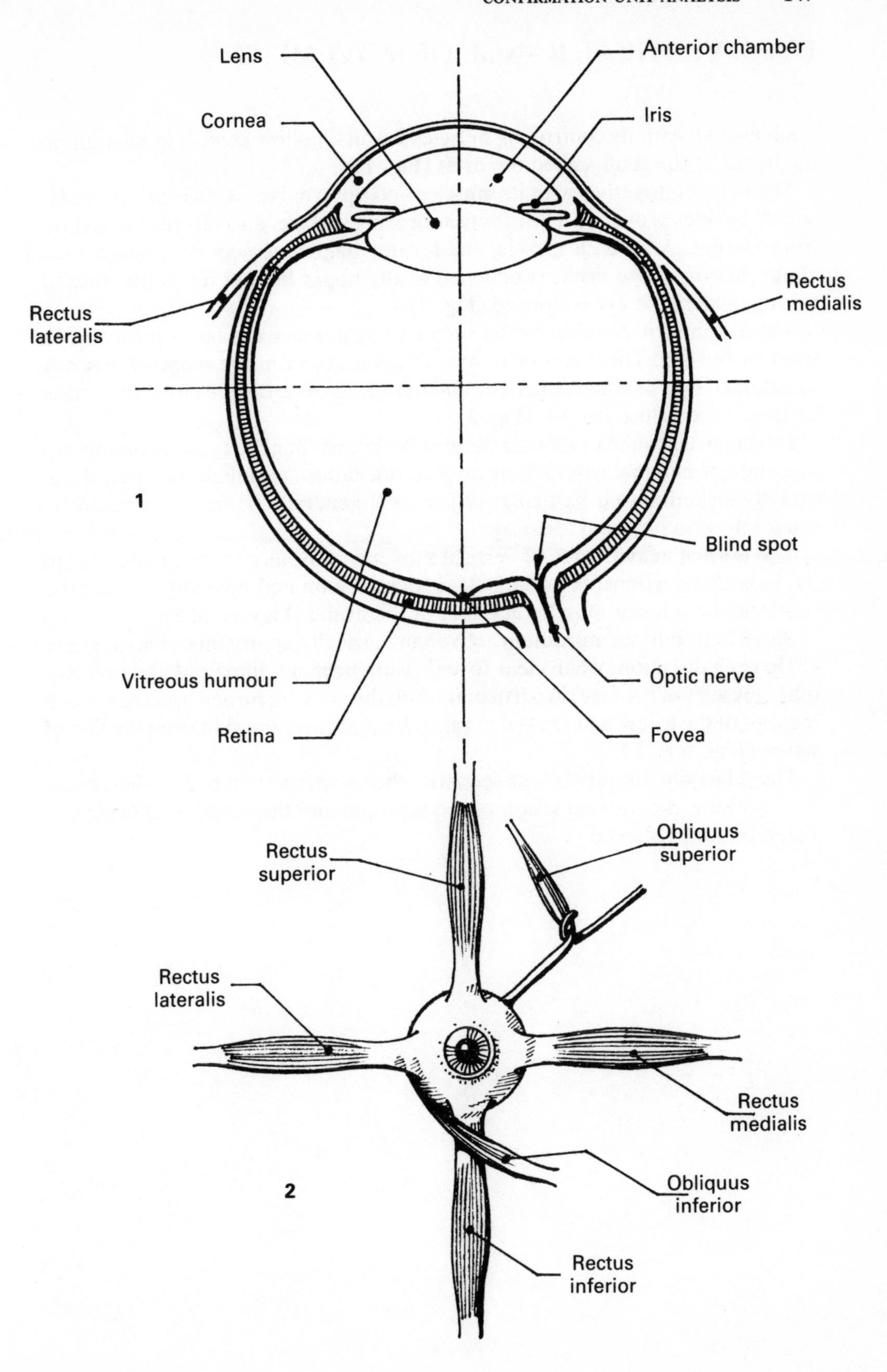
Lens
Anterior chamber
Cornea
Iris
Rectus medialis
Rectus lateralis
1
Blind spot
Vitreous humour
Optic nerve
Retina
Fovea
Rectus superior
Obliquus superior
Rectus lateralis
Rectus medialis
2
Obliquus inferior
Rectus inferior

EYES, VERTICAL RANGE OF MOVEMENT

Each eyeball with its controlling muscles lies in a hollow conical excavation in the bones of the skull, called the orbit (**Fig. 1**).

The eyeball, together with its muscles and optic nerve, is surrounded by fat which, besides providing a low friction-bearing surface, also affords protection from jarring. A seventh muscle, the levator palpebrae superior, which runs along the top of the orbit, is attached to the upper lid and fulfils the duty of raising it when the eye is opened (**Fig. 2**).

The eye, held in position by the surrounding muscles and fat, is protected in front by the lids. These consist of movable folds of skin, the shape of which is maintained by a thin layer of gristle and muscle fibres arranged circularly; these by their action close the lids (**Fig. 3**).

During straight ahead viewing the muscles controlling the eye movements are in a state of minimal contraction close to relaxation, although the eyes, if not visually locked onto a particular object, will generally be moved constantly, randomly searching and focusing.

The normal active range of vertical movement usually approximates 25° to 30° in both directions, providing clear foveal vision and involving mainly the superior and inferior muscles and that of the eyelid (**Figs 4** and **5**).

Movement into the maximum active range usually approximates an angle of 45° in each direction, when clear foveal vision becomes impaired and involves other muscles of the face, in particular when the eyes are turned upwards, when muscles of the forehead are used to raise the eyebrows and skin from the line of vision (**Figs. 6** and **7**).

These last situations are those seen with the two archers on p. 145, Figs. 6 and 7, and where clear foveal vision of the sight pin and the target is difficult and vision becomes blurred.

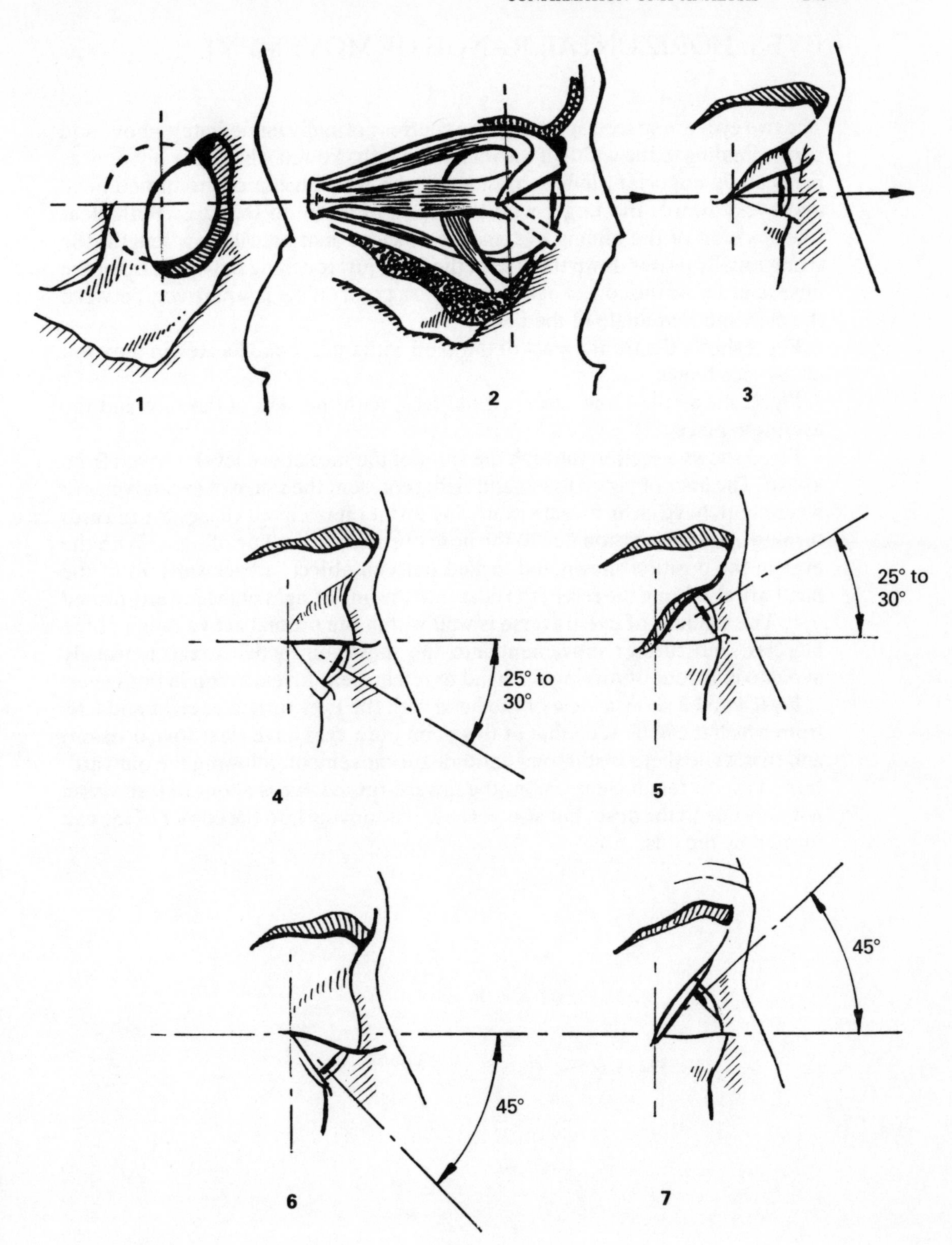
1
2
3
4
25° to
30°
5
25° to
30°
6
45°
7
45°

EYES, HORIZONTAL RANGE OF MOVEMENT

The two eyes are spaced apart with the centres normally immediately above and corresponding to the width of the relaxed mouth, a point which may not appear particularly important unless considering the relationship of the turned head and eyes towards the target with the string location on the face. With clear foveal vision of the aiming eye and an efficient anatomical draw length, the string usually passes down the side of the face, just touching the inside tip of the nose, and across the corner of the mouth to a point on the jaw part-way between the chin and rear angle of the jaw.

Fig. 1 shows the front aspect of the skull with the eyeball located in the orbit of the face bones.

Fig. 2 shows the same aspect of the face, with the skin of the face and the eyelids in place.

Fig. 3 shows a section through the front of the face at eye level, viewed from above. The lines of vision to left and right represent the range of eye movement where both have clear foveal vision; any further movement causes the inward-turning eye to lose vision due to the nose obstructing the line of sight. With the eyes in the position shown and locked onto an object, a backward tilt of the head will also bring the rest of the nose into the line of sight of the inward-turned eye. This amount of eye traverse is well within the normal active range of the muscles, and further movement into the maximum active range is usually avoided in favour of turning the head to retain clear foveal vision in both eyes.

Figs. 4 and **5** show a view of the head with the eyes turned to right and left, from which it can be seen that at this point both eyes have clear foveal vision, and that while there is still some latitude for movement, allowing the outward-turned eye to retain clear vision, the inward-turned eye is about to lose vision not only due to the nose, but also because it is moving into the corner of the eye formed by the lids.

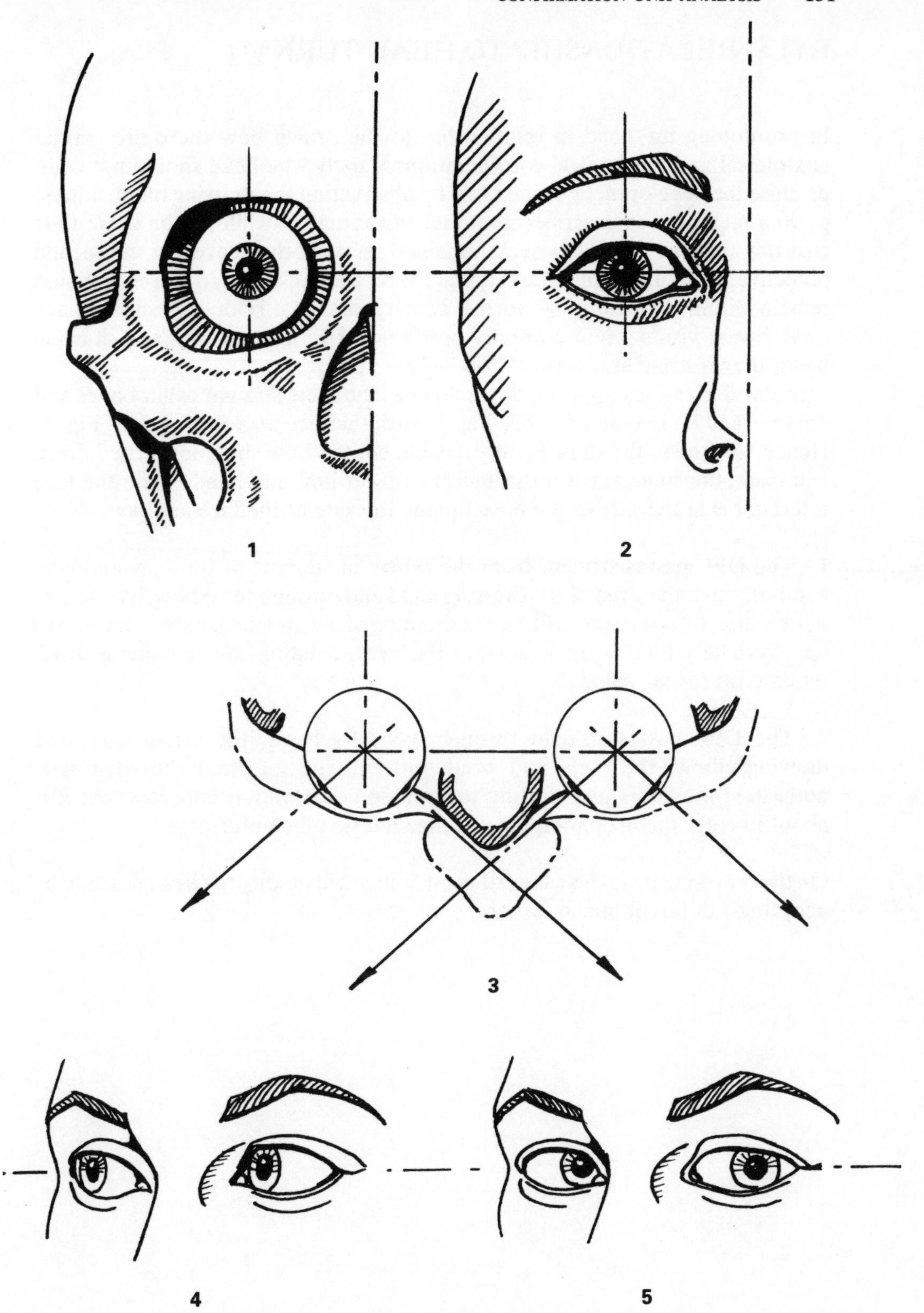
1
2
3
4
5

EYES, RELATIONSHIP TO HEAD TURN (1)

In positioning the head in relationship to the drawn bow there are certain anatomical and mechanical considerations. Firstly, the head should not compromise the development of the draw by obstructing the drawing hand, and on p. 96 a method was described that met this criterion while at the same time ensuring that the head and neck remained relaxed, thus covering the second objective. The third requirement is that the rotation of the head and eyes should remain within their range of normal activity, and that both eyes should have clear foveal vision when correctly positioned and aligned with the drawing hand, drawn string and vertical bow sight.

In the illustrations opposite the archer has the same straight collar bones and long-necked body type of p. 83, Fig. 1, with the face angles of p. 145, Fig. 3. Hence, as shown, the draw is fully developed, the bow shoulder settled down and back, the spine vertical through the power unit and head, while the face reference is at the side of the nose tip and the side of the face and jaw.

1 The DFL passes straight from the centre of support of the bow and bow hand, through the wrist of the drawing hand and through the elbow. The line of sight is directly above the DFL in the shooting plane and the head has rotated to approximately fifty degrees, so that the eyes, rotating the remaining forty, retain clear foveal vision.

2 The DFL passes straight through bow/bow hand, the arrow nock and drawing elbow, the body and head upright. The fact that the right sternomastoid muscle is just starting to show some definition indicates that it is about to enter the maximum active range but is still comfortable.

On the following page this same efficient archer will modify the head position by adopting a different face reference.

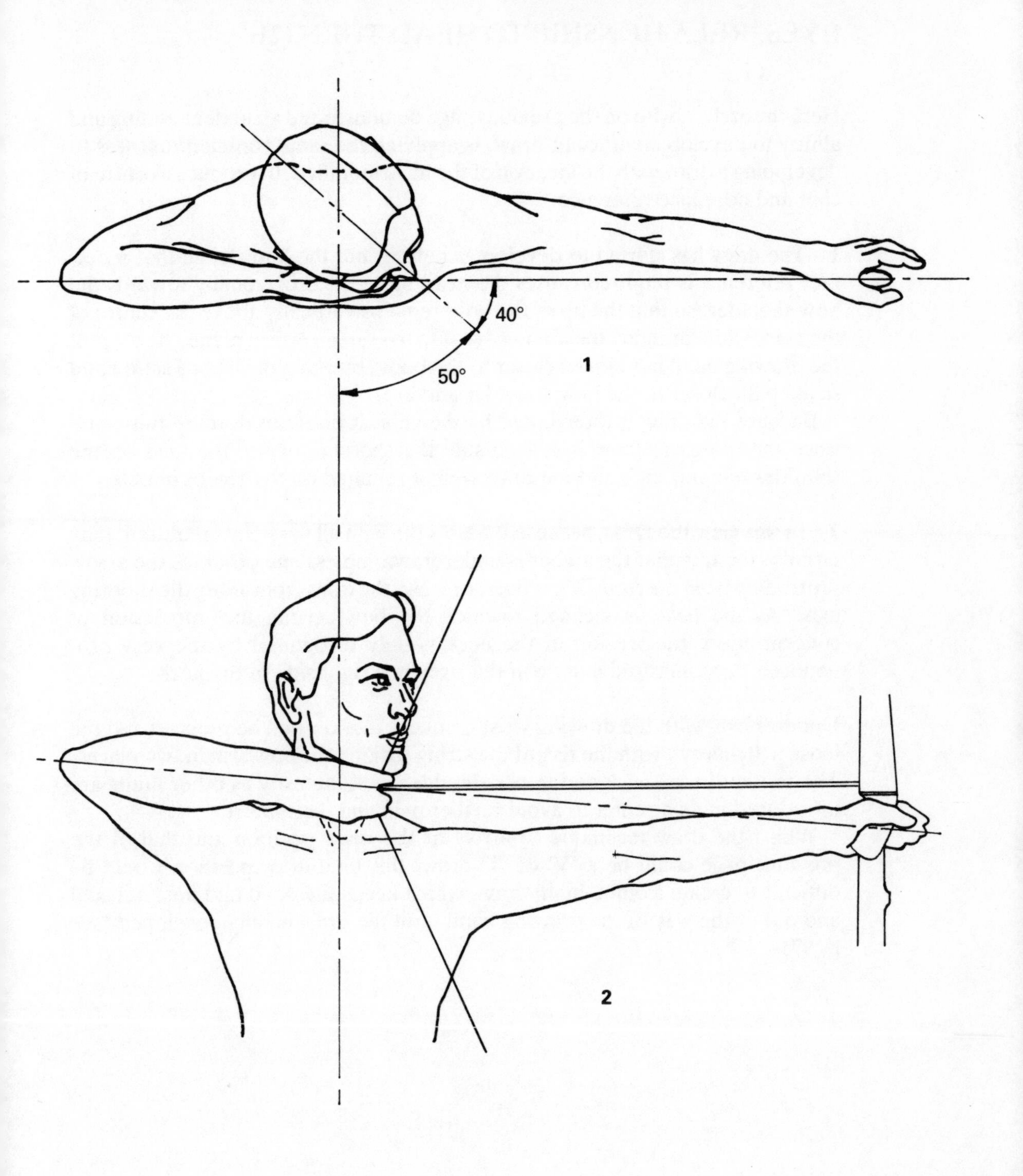
40°
50°
1
2

EYES, RELATIONSHIP TO HEAD TURN (2)

Here the archer, who on the previous page demonstrated an understanding and ability to develop an efficient draw, is applying the same conscientiousness to developing a draw with the location of the head modified, to produce a centre of chin and nose face reference.

1 The draw has started to develop as before, but the knowledge that a new face reference is required causes the head to be tilted diagonally towards the bow shoulder, so that the tip of the nose remains vertically above the centre of the chin, while bringing the aiming eye into the same vertical plane. As a result the drawing hand has moved closer to the body, bringing the line of action and string path closer to the bow shoulder and arm.

Because the draw is interrupted by the chin, it does not develop fully, and since the drawing elbow is still outside the shooting plane, the load on the shoulder remains high and the draw weight retained on the biceps muscle.

2 In this view the DFL, because it passes through all the points required, may disguise the fact that the archer is underdrawn, unless one observes the arrow protruding from the front of the riser, or views the draw from along the shooting axis. As the head is inclined towards the bow, giving the impression of concentration, the tension in the neck is only recognised by the very pronounced sternomastoid muscle in the stretched right side of the neck.

Underdrawn, with the drawing wrist cranked, the cast will be reduced and the loose a 'fly-away', with the risk of the string striking the bow arm in two places. The tension in the neck and upper shoulders will intensify as other faults are introduced in an attempt to avoid further pain and discomfort.

Whilst the draw technique to arrive at this draw position and that of the previous page could be a 'V' or 'T' draw, this final draw position would be difficult to create from a 'high' draw, which keeps the head and neck relaxed and out of the way of the drawing hand until the draw is fully developed (see p. 97).

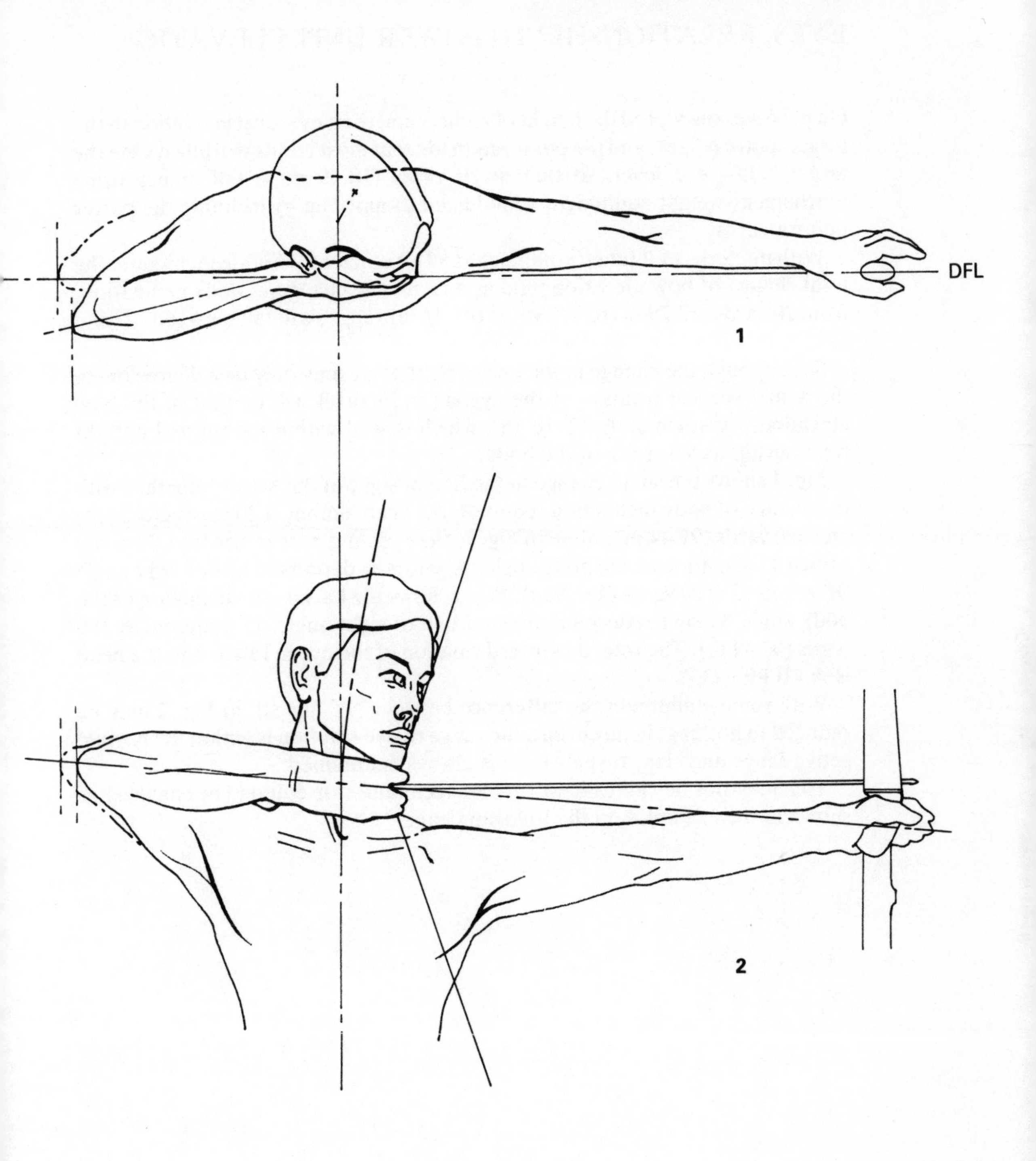
DFL
1
2

EYES, RELATIONSHIP TO POWER UNIT ELEVATION

On p. 66 we considered the height of archers and their eye level in relation to the target centre height, and the point was made that most adults will always see the target below eye level, so that at 20 yards (18.29 m) a tall archer using tournament-weight equipment would need to unit-aim by inclining the power unit forwards.

With modern, well tuned equipment and an efficient shooting technique, the total change of bow elevation, and as a result the change in body inclination, from 20 yards (18.29 m) to 100 yards (91.44 m) range, will fall between 12° and 15°.

So, although the change in the line of sight angle may only be a degree or so, the actual vertical rotation of the eyeball in its orbit will be that of the bow elevation, approximately 12° to 15°, which is well within the normal upright relationship to the trunk of the body.

Fig. 1 shows the small change in the line of sight to the target, together with the change of body inclination required, between aiming at 20 yards (18.29 m) and 100 yards (91.44 m), while in **Fig. 2**, the eyes and nose of the face show the forward inclination of the body angle 'A' with the depressed line of sight angle 'B' required at 20 yards (18.29 m). **Fig. 3** shows the backward inclination of the body angle 'C' and reduced depressed line of sight angle 'D' required at 100 yards (91.44 m). The total downward rotation of the eye in relation to the head is A+B+C−D.

With some equipment the difference between 'A' and 'B' in **Fig. 2** may be reduced to nothing; in any event, the range of eye rotation is within the normal active range and clear foveal vision is always maintained.

This may not be the case with other techniques or equipment changes, as shown in the examples on the following page.

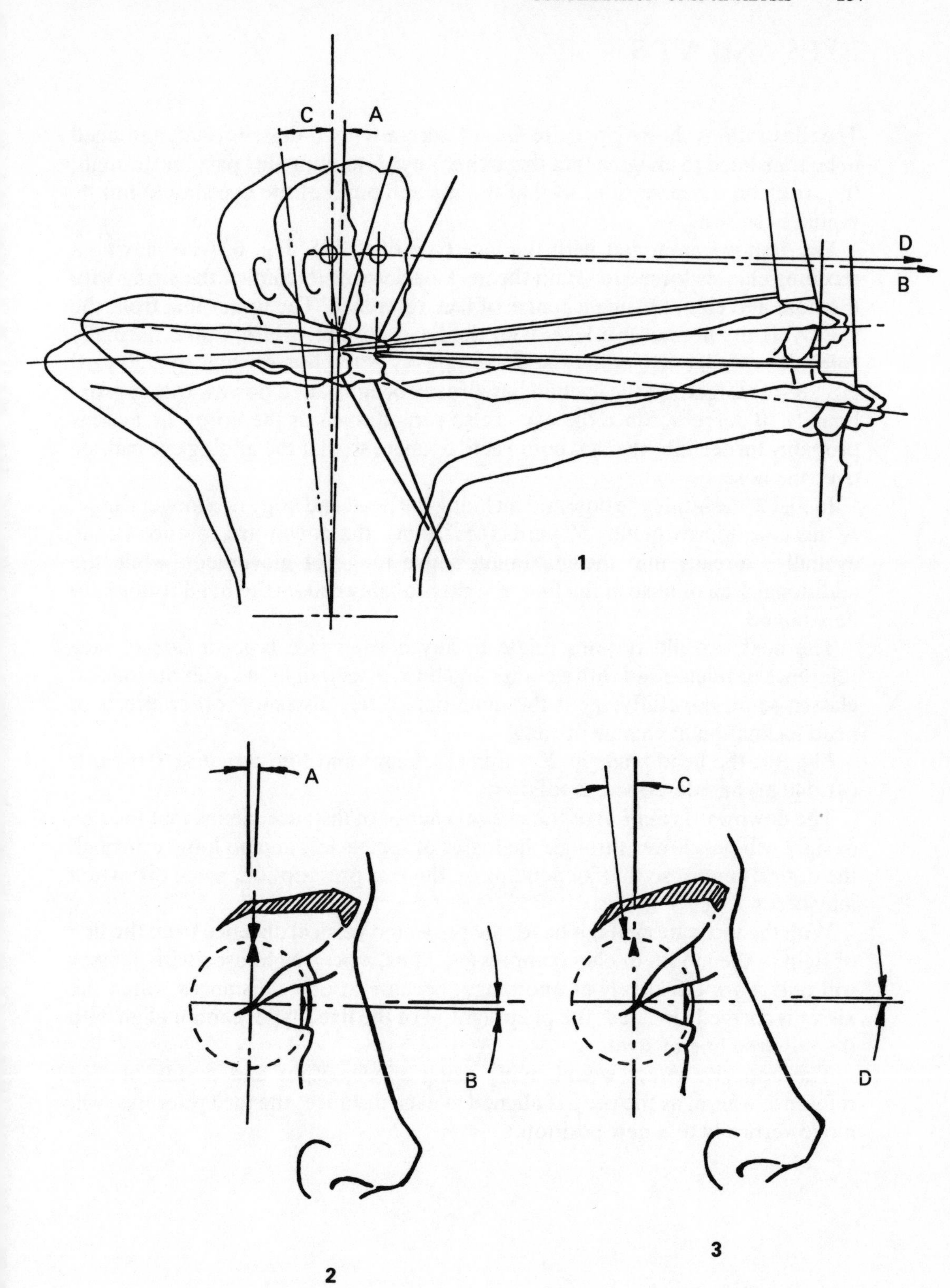
C
A
D
B
1
A
C
B
D
2
3

EYES AND AIDS

The illustrations shown opposite are, of necessity, two-dimensional, and need to be translated to imagine that the archer's eye is looking just past, or through, the string on the nose side, so that the iris and pupil of the eye should not be visible as shown.

Fig. 1 shows an archer with the face type of p. 145, Fig. 6, who, having a receding chin, is forced to strain the neck backwards to contact the string with the nose and chin, if using a centre of face reference. The upper line from the eye 'A' is the normal eye level with the head upright, which would normally coincide with line 'B', while the lower line 'C' is the line of sight to a 20 yard (18.288 m) target. So the eyeball has already been rotated downwards approximately 10 degrees. Since the eye is also turned towards the nose, the head is probably turned into the maximum active range, so that the aiming eye can see over the nose.

In **Fig. 2**, elevating the bow and inclining the head and body to a longer range, in this case approximately 50 yards (45.720 m), the downward rotation of the eyeball is already into the maximum active range of movement, while the additional area of nose in the line of sight probably causes the head rotation to be strained.

The next two illustrations relate to any normal face type, a side of face reference or release-aid with a compound bow, a peep sight, a kisser button and glasses—not, hopefully, all at the same time. They also show other effects of head inclination at change of range.

Fig. 3 is the head angle at 20 yards (18.288m) and **Fig. 4** that at 100 yards (91.440 m) and described as follows:

The downward rotation of the eyes at change of distance means that the line of sight will pass lower through the lenses of spectacles, and no longer through the optical centre, so that, depending on the lens prescription, some distortion may occur.

With the inclination of the head, the projected vertical distance from the line of sight to the mouth or chin compresses. Thus, a peep sight used with a kisser will only work effectively at one range, because at other distances, when the kisser is correctly located, the peep sight, if of the fixed type, cannot align with the required line of sight.

The opposite effect would apply using a peep sight and a side of face reference where, as the peep is aligned at each distance, the face reference will move vertically to a new position.

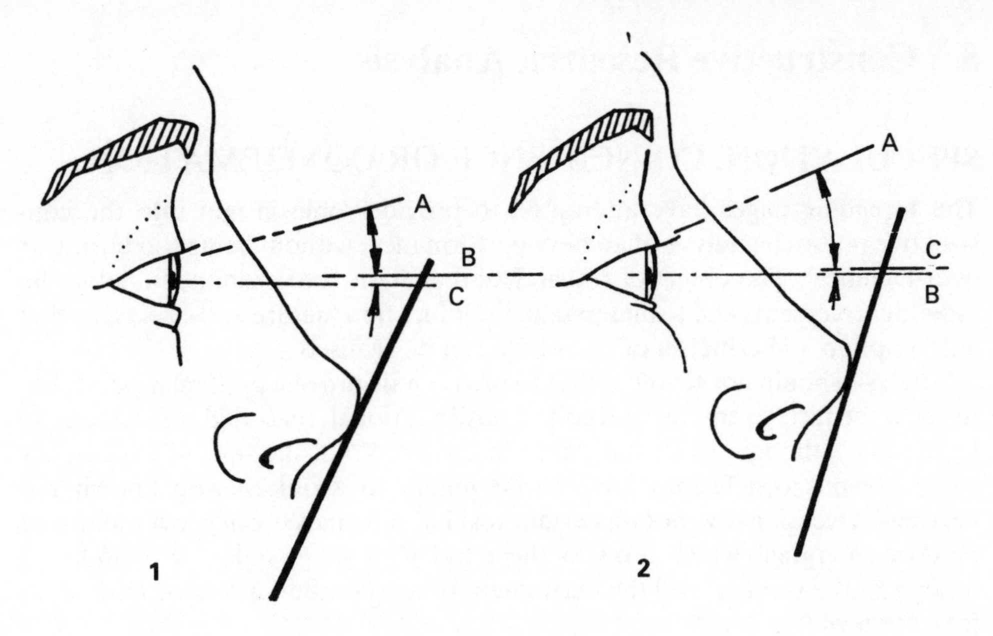
A
B
C
1
A
C
B
2

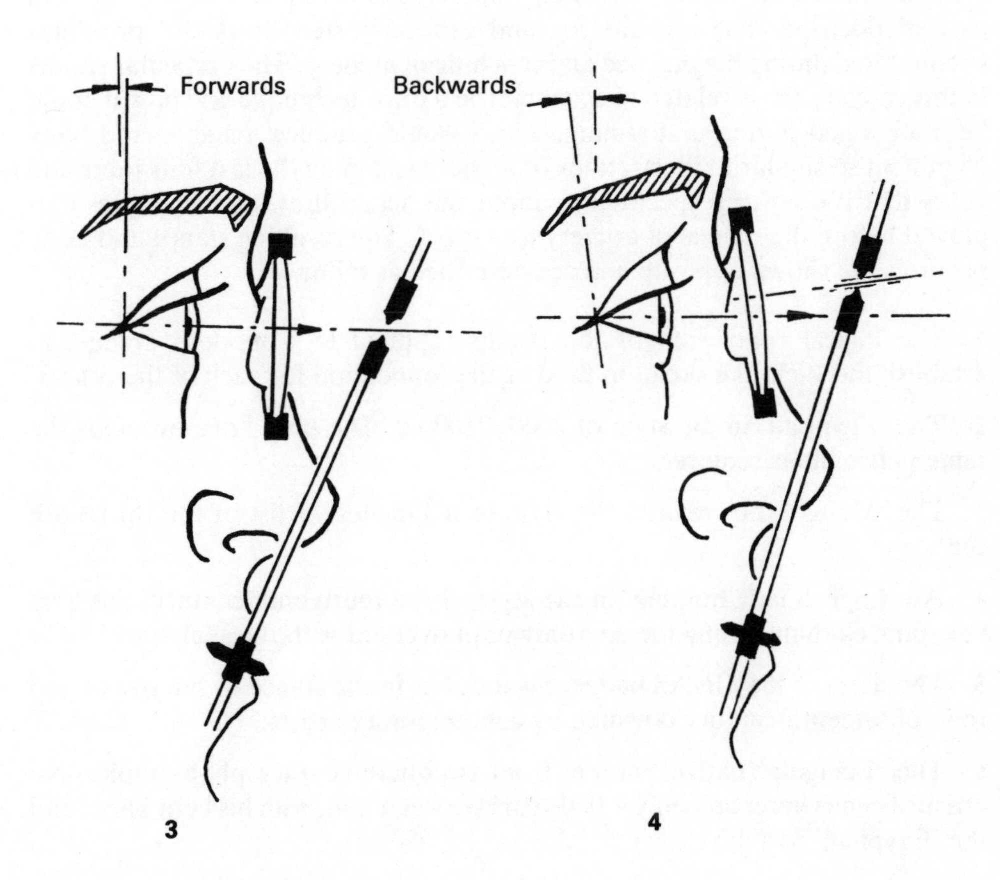
Forwards
Backwards
3
4

8 Constructive Research Analysis

SPECULATION, COINCIDENCE OR CONFIRMATION

The foregoing pages have attempted to provide some insight into the constructive research analysis of archery performance, without being too boring or over-technical. The object of research and analysis is to examine in detail the individual elements and to understand their function, nature and effects, so that a description and criticism of the whole can be realised.

Analysis should not set out either to prove or disprove a particular point, but to allow the facts to emerge and collect until a rational, reasoned conclusion can be made—although, as we have seen in this book, for the sake of expediency some obvious conclusions have to be made, to avoid chasing known red herrings. Occasionally, noting certain results, the analyst can see a picture or pattern emerging, which links in the mind with other older or abandoned aspects of the subject, and the excitement of a realisation has to be curbed, at least for a while.

Such a situation occurred during the mathematical modelling and creation of the illustrations for this book, when some results emerged that conflict with current doctrine, but account for and are supported by actual problems encountered during the practice and coaching of archery. The particular results in this case are those related to a symmetrical draw technique and how it could be maintained during unit-aiming, which would produce a stance and body alignment so similar to illustrations of archery spanning the last four thousand years that it opens up speculation about the actual drawing techniques employed before the revival of archery as a sport. The resulting stance and body postures are shown opposite and are described as follows:

1 The logical conclusion of the results, applied to a modern archer, to establish the stick-like skeleton used as the foundation for each of the others.

2 The 'Egyptian' in the style of 2000–2100 BC. The bent knee provides the same pelvic tilt as required.

3 The 'Mongol' bowman in the style of a Japanese artist of the thirteenth century.

4 An 'English lady hunting' in the style of the fourteenth century, the long sweeping clothing hiding the anatomy until overlaid with the skeleton.

5 The dress of the GNAS badge, maybe, but in the stance of the rows upon rows of fifteenth-century bowmen by contemporary artists.

6 The 'Liangula' native hunter, from twentieth-century photographs. No artistic licence here, and only 4,000 years between him, with his bent knee, and the 'Egyptian' with his.

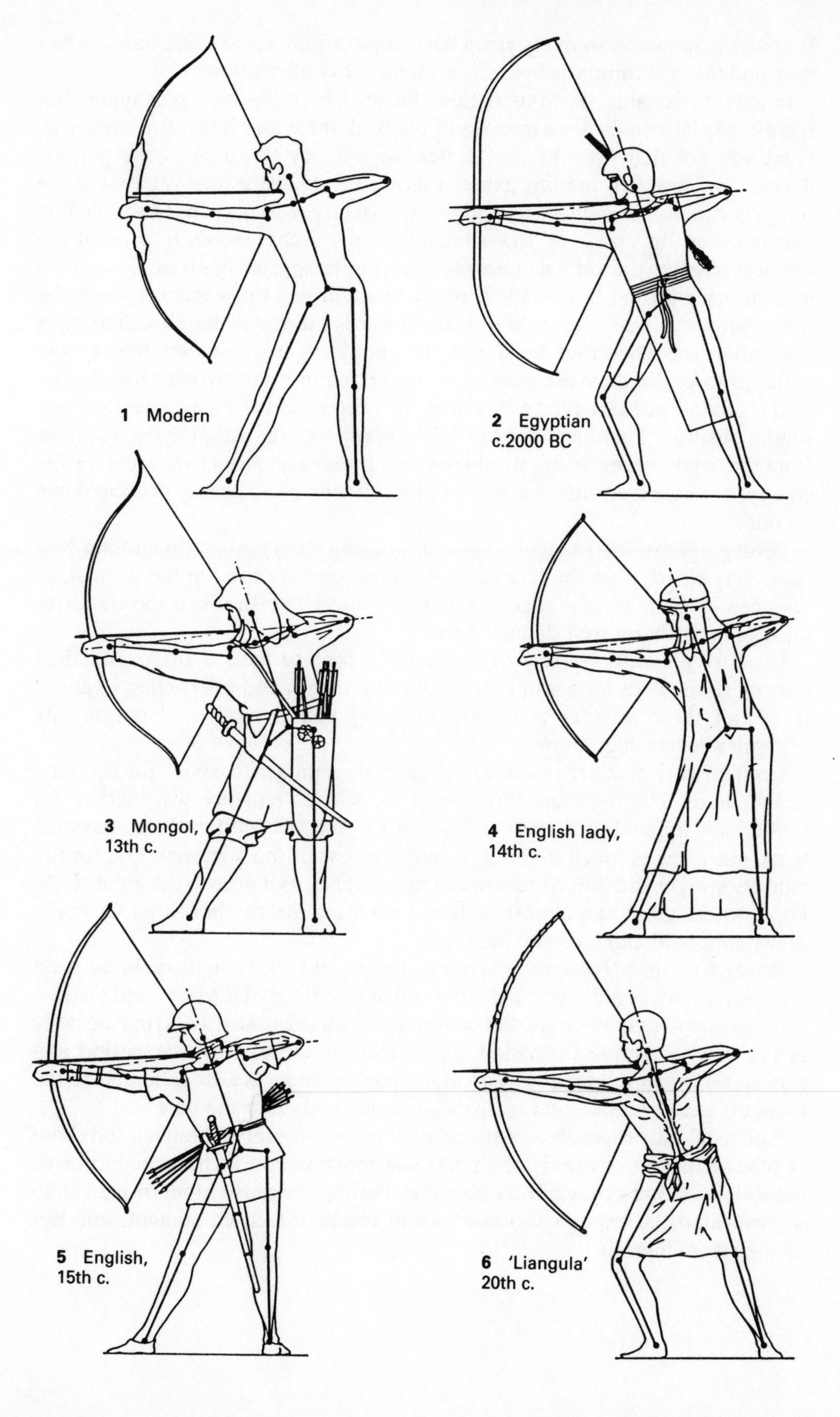
1 Modern
2 Egyptian
c.2000 BC
3 Mongol,
13th c.
4 English lady,
14th c.
5 English,
15th c.
6 'Liangula'
20th c.

War artists spanning so many years have depicted the same basic stance when they had the real thing to copy. Coincidence or confirmation?

It may reasonably be argued that the upright high-draw technique that recruits the latissimus dorsi muscles of the back throughout the draw development was not that used by the hunters or military bowmen of the periods illustrated. However, hunting game or facing an advancing enemy have certain things in common, totally unrelated to modern target archery, not least the fact that between the shots, or when reloading, the archer needs to present the smallest target to the animal or enemy. The hunter approaches from down wind in a crouch with the bow loaded, ready to stand and draw quickly when the target presents itself. The soldier leans towards the foe while reloading, thus presenting the armoured head and the shoulders as a smaller target, and certainly to load and loose arrows at any speed requires the arrows to be planted in the ground in front of the bowman, or presented for quick selection in a similar position. Standing upright while groping for and withdrawing an arrow from the belt or other device would not only present an attractive target for the enemy, but would do little for self-confidence seeing the enemy bearing down on one.

Photographs of the Liangula bowman drawing a very powerful hunting bow show very clearly that the latissimus dorsi muscles are used in the draw since they can be seen clearly, together with the lower two-thirds of the trapezius muscle, in the bare, well-defined back.

Experiments with leaning over the front foot to load a shaft, and then drawing as the body swings upright, prove that the up-and-over action required to recruit these muscles is remarkably easy and natural, and not readily recognisable as a high draw.

Until the revival of archery as a back garden, or parkland, sport, the shooting technique of standing erect throughout the whole sequence was neither described nor implied in earlier written works, and the modern basic shooting technique owes as much to the style and fashions of the Victorian era, for the military upright and timed sequence of movements, as it does to the great H. A. Ford, whose ghost can almost be heard counting the rhythm as pupils nock, draw, aim, hold and loose by numbers.

Roger Ascham's *Toxophilus* is not technical, but a lot can be deduced from his observations of archers at the butts and descriptions of the bows and arrows, while expressions in his and other contemporary works, such as 'laying the body in the bow', describe the visual appearance of archers, of that period and earlier, far better than that of Victorian times or since, the exception being the Liangula native hunter who really is laying his body into the bow.

Above all, and regardless of speculation about ancient techniques and those of other nations or periods, the point still remains that archery should be as natural, easy and enjoyable as possible. Perhaps because modern man is so sophisticated, he expects too much from the high-tech equipment, and not enough from himself.

The Last End

The majority of archery organisations at all levels, coaching groups, coach training courses, examinations, training manuals, books and magazines, usually devote more time and space debating, arguing and describing the history, rules of shooting, handicap tables, etiquette, finance, insurance and politics of the sport than they devote to the skills and practice of archery itself.

Archery Anatomy very deliberately sets out to present the physical actions and reactions of the human anatomy and that of the equipment, as they are applied to the practice and acquisition of the psychophysical skill required to shoot good arrows from a bow. If it fails in this respect, it is because it has only touched upon a few of the biological and mechanical areas of the sport, and time alone will tell if this objective has been achieved.

Although the motivation for acquiring a high skill level at archery has changed, the fact that it has survived so long through history, and still attracts large numbers of recruits, would suggest that the perceived benefits of the sport are related to it being a healthy individual physical exercise with a high degree of atavism attached to it.

The fact that the turnover in club membership is fairly regular, in that many leave within a few seasons to be replaced by other new members at a similar rate, who in their turn leave, is perhaps due to the very reasons given at the top of this page—namely that more attention is paid to getting them shooting in tournaments, with all the associated problems of rules, handicaps and classifications, than to helping them attain a skill level at which archery becomes relatively easy and enjoyed at a psychophysical level. The additional burden of rules and regulations could then be taken on board without affecting the practice and development of higher competitive skills. The reasons for the emphasis on the non-physical or biological aspects of archery are easy to understand. The understanding of the man-made rules and regulations can be tested by set question-and-answer examination, while the examination of the creative ability to apply knowledge of basic anatomy and physics to the solution of unique problems, and to provide the correct solution, cannot be tested by a set examination and can only be assessed and evaluated by another with the same or similar intuitive ability.

Archery Anatomy, while it may provide some answers to some questions directly, aims to provide the raw material and incentive for the coach or performer to question why this or that happens when so and so does that. And having asked why, to work it out, analyse it, test it, prove it and then apply it. When dealing with the individual human body and mental-processing ability, there are no set questions and no set answers, for they are all as unique as the individual.

NOTE: The expression 'the last end' means the last arrows shot.